I0703610

VEGETARIAN HISTAMINE INTOLERANCE COOKBOOK

Nutritious and Tasty Low-Reaction Cuisine

Sophia j. Smith

Copyright © 2024 [SOPHIA J. SMITH]

All rights reserved. No part of this material may be reproduced, distributed, or transmitted in any form or by any means, including photocopying, recording, or other electronic or mechanical methods, without the prior written permission of the copyright owner, except in the case of brief quotations embodied in critical reviews and certain other noncommercial uses permitted by copyright law.

INTRODUCTION

Welcome to the "Vegetarian Histamine Intolerance Cookbook," a culinary guide dedicated to those navigating the challenging waters of histamine intolerance while maintaining a vegetarian lifestyle. This book is crafted with care and expertise to help you enjoy delicious, nutritious meals without the worry of triggering histamine-related symptoms.

Histamine intolerance can be a complex and often misunderstood condition, affecting many aspects of daily life, including diet. High-histamine foods can lead to various symptoms, from headaches and digestive issues to skin reactions and more. Managing these symptoms through diet is crucial, and this can be particularly challenging for vegetarians, as many common vegetarian staples are high in histamines.

This cookbook aims to bridge the gap, offering a variety of recipes that are both low in histamines and full of flavor. Whether you are newly diagnosed or have been managing histamine intolerance for years, you will find an array of options to suit your tastes and dietary needs. From vibrant breakfasts and hearty lunches to satisfying dinners and delightful desserts, this cookbook provides a comprehensive guide to eating well while living with histamine intolerance.

We begin with a foundational understanding of histamine intolerance, exploring its symptoms, causes, and the critical role of diet in managing this condition. Following this, we delve into the benefits of a vegetarian diet and how it can be harmoniously integrated with histamine intolerance management. Essential tips for stocking your kitchen and planning your meals will empower you to make informed and healthful choices every day.

Each recipe in this book is designed with care, emphasizing fresh, wholesome ingredients that are naturally low in histamines. You'll discover creative ways to prepare familiar favorites and new dishes that will become staples in your culinary repertoire. We have also included valuable nutritional information and practical tips for dining out, ensuring that you can maintain your diet with confidence and ease, even outside of your home.

Living with histamine intolerance does not mean sacrificing taste or variety. With the right knowledge and recipes, you can enjoy a diverse and satisfying vegetarian diet. This cookbook is your companion on this journey, providing the tools and inspiration you need to thrive.

We hope that this collection of recipes brings joy, health, and delicious flavors to your table. Welcome to a world of vibrant, low-histamine, vegetarian cuisine!

TABLE OF CONTENTS

1. Understanding Histamine Intolerance

1.1 What is Histamine?

Histamine is a naturally occurring compound that plays a vital role in the body's immune response, digestion, and central nervous system. It is a biogenic amine, which means it is derived from an amino acid—in this case, histidine. Histamine is involved in several critical functions:

1. Immune Response:
Histamine is a key player in the body's defense mechanism against allergens and infections. It is released by mast cells and basophils (types of white blood cells) when the immune system detects a foreign invader. This release causes blood vessels to dilate and become more permeable, allowing other immune cells to reach the site of infection or injury more quickly.

2. Gastrointestinal Function:
In the digestive system, histamine helps regulate the secretion of gastric acid in the stomach, which is essential for breaking down food and absorbing nutrients. Histamine produced in the stomach binds to H2 receptors on parietal cells, stimulating the production of gastric acid.

3. Neurotransmission:
Histamine acts as a neurotransmitter in the brain, influencing various functions such as wakefulness, appetite, and cognitive processes. It helps regulate the sleep-wake cycle and is involved in the body's response to stress.

Despite its crucial roles, an excess of histamine can lead to adverse reactions, particularly in individuals with histamine intolerance. Normally, the enzyme diamine oxidase

(DAO) breaks down histamine in the digestive tract, while histamine N-methyltransferase (HNMT) does so in other tissues. However, if these enzymes are deficient or overwhelmed, histamine accumulates, causing symptoms.

Understanding histamine and its role in the body is the first step in managing histamine intolerance. In the next sections, we will delve deeper into the symptoms and diagnosis, explore the causes and triggers, and discuss how dietary adjustments can help manage this condition effectively.

1.2 Symptoms and Diagnosis

Histamine intolerance can present a complex array of symptoms that often overlap with other conditions, making it challenging to diagnose. Recognizing these symptoms and understanding the diagnostic process is essential for effective management.

Symptoms of Histamine Intolerance:

Histamine intolerance symptoms can affect various body systems, leading to a wide range of clinical presentations. The seriousness and mix of side effects can change from one individual to another.

1. Gastrointestinal Symptoms:

- Bloating: Excess histamine can cause the stomach and intestines to produce more acid, leading to discomfort and bloating.
- Diarrhea: Increased histamine levels can accelerate intestinal motility, resulting in loose stools or diarrhea.
- Stomach Cramps: Histamine can trigger spasms in the gastrointestinal tract, causing abdominal pain and cramps.

2. Respiratory Symptoms:

- Nasal Congestion: Histamine can cause the nasal passages to swell, leading to stuffiness and congestion.
- Sneezing: Excess histamine can irritate the nasal passages, causing frequent sneezing.
- Asthma-like Symptoms: In some individuals, histamine can cause bronchoconstriction, leading to wheezing and shortness of breath.

3. Skin Symptoms:

- Hives (Urticaria): Raised, itchy welts on the skin can occur as a direct result of histamine release.
- Itching: Generalized itching, particularly in response to consuming high-histamine foods.
- Flushing: Reddening of the skin, especially on the face and chest, often accompanies histamine release.

4. Cardiovascular Symptoms:

- Headaches or Migraines: Histamine can dilate blood vessels in the brain, leading to headaches or migraines.
- Hypertension: Increased histamine can cause elevated blood pressure in some individuals.
- Irregular Heart Rate: Histamine can affect heart rate and rhythm, sometimes causing palpitations.

5. Neurological and Psychological Symptoms:

- Fatigue: Chronic histamine intolerance can lead to persistent tiredness and fatigue.
- Dizziness: Histamine can affect blood pressure and circulation, causing dizziness or lightheadedness.
- Anxiety or Panic Attacks: Elevated histamine levels can influence neurotransmitter function, leading to anxiety and panic attacks.

Diagnosis of Histamine Intolerance:

Diagnosing histamine intolerance can be complex due to the non-specific nature of the symptoms and their overlap with other conditions such as allergies, food intolerances, and gastrointestinal disorders. The accompanying advances are commonly engaged with the demonstrative cycle:

1. Clinical Evaluation:

- Medical History: A thorough medical history is essential, focusing on the patient's symptoms, dietary habits, and any relevant family history.
- Symptom Diary: Keeping a detailed symptom diary that includes food intake, symptoms, and timing can help identify patterns and potential triggers.

2. Dietary Assessment:

- Elimination Diet: This involves removing high-histamine foods from the diet for a specific period (typically 2-4 weeks) and monitoring symptom changes. Improvement during this phase suggests histamine intolerance.
- Challenge Test: After the elimination phase, high-histamine foods are gradually reintroduced to see if symptoms recur, confirming the diagnosis.

3. Laboratory Tests:

- DAO Enzyme Activity Test: This test measures the activity of diamine oxidase (DAO), the enzyme responsible for breaking down histamine in the gut. Low DAO activity indicates a potential histamine intolerance.
- Histamine Levels in Blood or Urine: Elevated histamine levels in blood or urine samples can support the diagnosis.
- Genetic Testing: Some individuals may undergo genetic testing to identify mutations affecting DAO or other related enzymes.

4. Exclusion of Other Conditions:

- Allergy Testing: Skin prick tests or specific IgE blood tests can rule out true food allergies.

- Gastrointestinal Evaluation: Endoscopy, colonoscopy, or tests for conditions like celiac disease, irritable bowel syndrome (IBS), or small intestinal bacterial overgrowth (SIBO) can exclude other causes of gastrointestinal symptoms.

Histamine intolerance manifests through a variety of symptoms that can impact multiple body systems. Due to the complexity of the condition, a comprehensive approach combining clinical evaluation, dietary assessment, and laboratory tests is necessary for an accurate diagnosis. Understanding these symptoms and the diagnostic process is crucial for managing histamine intolerance effectively and improving quality of life. In the following sections, we will explore the causes and triggers of histamine intolerance and how dietary adjustments can help manage this condition.

1.3 Causes and Triggers

Histamine intolerance arises from an imbalance between histamine intake and the body's ability to break it down. Several factors contribute to this condition, and identifying these causes and triggers is crucial for managing symptoms effectively.

Causes of Histamine Intolerance:

1. Enzyme Deficiency:

- Diamine Oxidase (DAO) Deficiency: DAO is the primary enzyme responsible for breaking down histamine in the digestive tract. A deficiency in DAO can lead to the accumulation of histamine, resulting in intolerance. Factors such as genetics, gastrointestinal diseases, or medications can impair DAO activity.
- Histamine N-Methyltransferase (HNMT) Deficiency: HNMT is another enzyme involved in histamine breakdown, particularly in the liver and other tissues. While less commonly implicated than DAO, deficiencies in HNMT can also contribute to histamine intolerance.

2. Genetic Factors:

- Genetic mutations can affect the production and function of DAO and HNMT enzymes, making some individuals more susceptible to histamine intolerance. These genetic variations can be inherited and may explain familial patterns of the condition.

3. Gut Health and Microbiota:

- The gut microbiota plays a significant role in histamine metabolism. Dysbiosis, an imbalance in the gut microbiota, can increase histamine production or decrease its breakdown, leading to intolerance. Conditions like small intestinal bacterial overgrowth (SIBO) and leaky gut syndrome can exacerbate this problem.

4. Chronic Diseases:

- Chronic conditions such as inflammatory bowel disease (IBD), irritable bowel syndrome (IBS), and celiac disease can damage the gut lining and impair DAO production, contributing to histamine intolerance.

5. Medications:

- Certain medications can inhibit DAO activity or increase histamine release. Common culprits include non-steroidal anti-inflammatory drugs (NSAIDs), antibiotics, antidepressants, and antihypertensive medications. These drugs can disrupt histamine metabolism and exacerbate symptoms.

Triggers of Histamine Intolerance:

Identifying and avoiding triggers is essential for managing histamine intolerance. Triggers can vary widely among individuals, but common categories include:

1. Dietary Triggers:

- High-Histamine Foods: Certain foods naturally contain high levels of histamine or can stimulate histamine release in the body. Common high-histamine foods include aged cheeses, fermented foods (such as sauerkraut and yogurt), processed meats (like salami and sausage), alcohol (especially red wine and beer), and certain fish (such as tuna and mackerel).
- Histamine Liberators: Some foods do not contain high levels of histamine but can cause the body to release histamine. Examples include strawberries, tomatoes, chocolate, nuts, and certain spices.

- Food Additives: Additives and preservatives, such as sulfites, benzoates, and artificial colorings, can trigger histamine release in sensitive individuals.

2. Environmental Triggers:

- Allergens: Exposure to environmental allergens such as pollen, dust mites, and animal dander can increase histamine levels in the body, exacerbating symptoms.
- Insect Bites and Stings: Insect bites or stings can cause localized histamine release, leading to swelling and itching.

3. Lifestyle Triggers:

- Stress: Chronic stress can affect the immune system and gut health, leading to increased histamine production or decreased breakdown.
- Exercise: Intense physical activity can sometimes trigger histamine release, especially in individuals with histamine intolerance. Moderate exercise is generally beneficial, but it's important to listen to your body and avoid overexertion.
- Temperature Changes: Rapid changes in temperature, such as moving from a hot environment to a cold one, can trigger histamine release in some individuals.

4. Hormonal Changes:

- Hormonal fluctuations, particularly those related to the menstrual cycle, can influence histamine levels. Some women may experience heightened symptoms of histamine intolerance during certain phases of their cycle.

1.4 The Role of Diet in Managing Histamine Intolerance

Diet plays a critical role in managing histamine intolerance. Since histamine is present in many foods and can be influenced by dietary choices, careful meal planning and food selection are essential for reducing symptoms and improving quality of life.

Understanding Low-Histamine Diets:

A low-histamine diet involves avoiding foods that are high in histamine or that trigger histamine release in the body. It also focuses on incorporating foods that are low in histamine and supportive of overall gut health.

High-Histamine Foods to Avoid:

1. Aged and Fermented Foods:

Cheeses: Aged cheeses such as cheddar, Parmesan, and blue cheese contain high levels of histamine.
Fermented Products: Sauerkraut, kimchi, soy sauce, miso, and pickled vegetables are rich in histamine.
Alcoholic Beverages: Wine, beer, and champagne can increase histamine levels.
2. Processed and Preserved Foods:

Processed Meats: Salami, ham, bacon, and sausages are high in histamine due to curing and processing.
Canned and Smoked Fish: Tuna, mackerel, and sardines in cans, as well as smoked fish, should be avoided.
3. Certain Vegetables and Fruits:

Nightshades: Tomatoes, eggplants, and peppers can trigger histamine release.

Certain Fruits: Strawberries, avocados, bananas, and citrus fruits may also release histamine.

4. Other Triggers:

Chocolate and Cocoa: These can stimulate histamine release.

Vinegar and Foods Containing Vinegar: Salad dressings, ketchup, and pickles are examples.

Dietary Strategies for Managing Histamine Intolerance:

1. Freshness is Key:

Consume foods as fresh as possible. Histamine levels increase in foods as they age, so avoid leftovers and choose fresh produce, meats, and dairy alternatives.

2. Food Preparation:

Pick straightforward cooking strategies, for example, steaming, bubbling, or barbecuing. Avoid slow-cooking or fermenting, which can increase histamine levels.

3. Personalized Diet:

Histamine intolerance can vary widely among individuals. Keeping a food diary and noting any reactions can help identify personal triggers and safe foods.

4. Hydration:

Staying well-hydrated supports overall health and helps the body manage histamine levels. Drink plenty of water throughout the day.

5. Probiotics and Gut Health:

Probiotic supplements and prebiotic-rich foods can support a healthy gut microbiome, which may help in managing histamine levels. Choose probiotics that do not contain histamine-producing strains.

Supplements and Nutrients to Support Histamine Breakdown:

1. DAO Supplements:

These supplements can help increase the body's ability to break down histamine, especially when taken before meals.

2. Vitamin C:

Vitamin C acts as a natural antihistamine and supports the immune system. Include vitamin C-rich foods like bell peppers, kiwi, and broccoli in your diet.

3. Vitamin B6:

This vitamin is essential for DAO enzyme function. Good sources include sunflower seeds, pistachios, and chickpeas.

4. Omega-3 Fatty Acids:

Anti-inflammatory omega-3s can help reduce histamine symptoms. Include sources like flaxseeds, chia seeds, and walnuts.

2. Embracing a Vegetarian Lifestyle

2.1 Benefits of a Vegetarian Diet

Adopting a vegetarian diet offers numerous health benefits, which can be particularly advantageous for individuals managing histamine intolerance. A vegetarian diet focuses on plant-based foods, which are typically lower in histamine and can help reduce symptoms associated with histamine intolerance. Here are some key benefits of a vegetarian diet:

1. Lower Histamine Levels:

Fresh Vegetables and Fruits: Vegetables and fruits are generally low in histamine, especially when consumed fresh. This reduces the risk of histamine buildup in the body, which can help alleviate symptoms.

Minimized Histamine Liberators: Many plant-based foods are less likely to trigger histamine release compared to animal products, particularly aged or processed meats.
2. Rich in Nutrients:

Vitamins and Minerals: A vegetarian diet is rich in essential vitamins and minerals, such as vitamin C, vitamin E, potassium, and magnesium. These nutrients support overall health and can help manage histamine levels.

Antioxidants: Fruits and vegetables are high in antioxidants, which combat oxidative stress and inflammation, potentially reducing histamine-related symptoms.

3. Improved Gut Health:

Fiber-Rich Foods: A vegetarian diet is high in dietary fiber, which supports a healthy digestive system by promoting regular bowel movements and maintaining gut flora balance.

Prebiotic Foods: Plant-based foods like garlic, onions, and asparagus are prebiotics that feed beneficial gut bacteria, supporting a healthy microbiome that can help regulate histamine levels.

4. Anti-Inflammatory Properties:

Omega-3 Fatty Acids: While fish is a common source of omega-3s, plant-based sources like flaxseeds, chia seeds, and walnuts provide these anti-inflammatory fatty acids without the high histamine content of certain fish.

Phytonutrients: Vegetables and fruits contain phytonutrients with anti-inflammatory properties, helping to reduce overall inflammation in the body, which can be beneficial for managing histamine intolerance.

5. Weight Management and Metabolic Health:

Lower Caloric Density: Vegetarian diets tend to be lower in calories while still providing ample nutrients, which can help with weight management.

Improved Metabolism: A balanced vegetarian diet can improve metabolic health by regulating blood sugar levels and enhancing insulin sensitivity.

6. Reduced Risk of Chronic Diseases:

Cardiovascular Health: A vegetarian diet is associated with a lower risk of cardiovascular diseases due to reduced intake of saturated fats and cholesterol and increased consumption of heart-healthy foods.

Lower Cancer Risk: Diets high in fruits and vegetables are linked to a reduced risk of certain cancers, including colon and breast cancer, due to their high fiber and antioxidant content.

7. Ethical and Environmental Benefits:

Animal Welfare: A vegetarian diet avoids the consumption of animal products, aligning with ethical considerations regarding animal welfare.

Environmental Impact: Plant-based diets have a lower environmental footprint, contributing to sustainability by reducing greenhouse gas emissions, deforestation, and water usage associated with animal farming.

2.2 Nutritional Considerations for Vegetarians

While a vegetarian diet offers numerous health benefits, it is important to ensure that all essential nutrients are adequately consumed. This is especially crucial for individuals with histamine intolerance, as they need to manage their condition while maintaining overall nutritional balance. Here are the key nutritional considerations for vegetarians:

1. Protein:

Sources: Plant-based protein sources include legumes (lentils, chickpeas, beans), tofu, tempeh, quinoa, nuts, seeds, and whole grains.

Amino Acids: It's essential to consume an assortment of protein sources to guarantee a total amino corrosive profile. Combining different plant proteins throughout the day can help achieve this balance.
2. Iron:

Sources: Good plant-based sources of iron include lentils, chickpeas, beans, tofu, spinach, pumpkin seeds, and fortified cereals.

Absorption: Non-heme iron from plant sources is less easily absorbed than heme iron from animal products. Consuming vitamin C-rich foods (such as bell peppers, broccoli, and citrus fruits) alongside iron-rich foods can enhance absorption.
3. Vitamin B12:

Sources: Vitamin B12 is basically tracked down in creature items. Vegetarians should consider fortified foods (such as plant-based milk, nutritional yeast, and breakfast cereals) and supplements to meet their needs.

Importance: B12 is crucial for nerve function and red blood cell production. Deficiency can lead to anemia and neurological issues.

4. Omega-3 Fatty Acids:

Sources: Plant-based sources of omega-3s include flaxseeds, chia seeds, hemp seeds, walnuts, and algae-based supplements.

Conversion: The body converts alpha-linolenic acid (ALA) from plant sources into the more active forms (EPA and DHA), but this process is not very efficient. Including a variety of ALA-rich foods and considering algae-based DHA supplements can help.

5. Calcium:

Sources: Non-dairy sources of calcium include fortified plant-based milk, tofu made with calcium sulfate, leafy greens (such as kale and bok choy), almonds, and sesame seeds.

Bone Health: Adequate calcium intake is essential for bone health. Vitamin D also plays a role in calcium absorption and should be considered in conjunction with calcium intake.

6. Vitamin D:

Sources: Sun exposure is a primary source of vitamin D. Dietary sources include fortified plant-based milk and supplements.

Importance: Vitamin D is important for bone health and immune function. Vegetarians, especially those living in areas with limited sunlight, should monitor their vitamin D levels and consider supplements if necessary.

7. Zinc:

Sources: Zinc-rich plant foods include legumes, chickpeas, lentils, seeds (pumpkin, sesame, and sunflower), nuts, whole grains, and fortified cereals.

Absorption: Phytates in plant foods can inhibit zinc absorption. Soaking, sprouting, and fermenting grains and legumes can reduce phytate levels and improve zinc absorption.

8. Iodine:

Sources: Iodine is found in iodized salt, sea vegetables (such as seaweed), and fortified foods.

Thyroid Function: Iodine is essential for thyroid function. Vegetarians should ensure they use iodized salt or consume sea vegetables regularly.

9. Protein Combining:

Combining Foods: While it's not necessary to combine proteins at every meal, ensuring a varied diet throughout the day helps achieve a complete amino acid profile. Examples include rice and beans, hummus and whole grain bread, and peanut butter on whole grain toast.

10. Phytonutrients:

Variety: Consuming a wide variety of colorful fruits and vegetables ensures an intake of diverse phytonutrients, which have antioxidant and anti-inflammatory properties beneficial for overall health.

Part I: Foundations of a Low-Histamine Vegetarian Diet

3. Pantry Essentials and Kitchen Tools

3.1 Stocking a Low-Histamine Kitchen

Stocking a low-histamine kitchen is crucial for managing histamine intolerance while maintaining a nutritious and varied vegetarian diet. This involves selecting fresh, minimally processed ingredients and having the right tools to prepare and store meals. Here's a comprehensive guide to stocking your kitchen with low-histamine essentials and the necessary tools:

Fresh and Frozen Vegetables:

- Leafy Greens: Spinach, kale, lettuce, Swiss chard
- Root Vegetables: Carrots, sweet potatoes, beets, parsnips
- Cruciferous Vegetables: Broccoli, cauliflower, cabbage
- Other Vegetables: Zucchini, cucumbers, bell peppers (green and yellow), green beans

Fresh and Frozen Fruits:

- Berries: Blueberries, raspberries, blackberries
- Other Fruits: Apples, pears, melons (watermelon, cantaloupe), peaches

Proteins:

- Legumes: Lentils, chickpeas, black beans, white beans
- Tofu and Tempeh: Ensure they are fresh and minimally processed
- Grains: Quinoa, amaranth, buckwheat

Grains and Seeds:

- Whole Grains: Rice (white and basmati), oats, millet, barley
- Seeds: Flaxseeds, chia seeds, hemp seeds, sunflower seeds
- Nuts: Almonds, walnuts, pecans (ensure they are fresh and unsalted)

Dairy Alternatives:

- Plant-Based Milks: Almond milk, rice milk, coconut milk (ensure they are unsweetened and free from additives)
- Nut Butters: Almond butter, sunflower seed butter (ensure they are fresh and free from additives)

Oils and Fats:

- Oils: Extra virgin olive oil, coconut oil, avocado oil, flaxseed oil
- Other Fats: Fresh avocados (if tolerated), ghee (if consuming dairy-free alternatives)

Herbs and Spices:

- Herbs: Fresh basil, parsley, cilantro, thyme, rosemary, oregano
- Spices: Turmeric, ginger, garlic (fresh or powdered), cumin, coriander

Condiments and Additives:

- Salt: Sea salt, Himalayan pink salt
- Natural Sweeteners: Raw honey, maple syrup (in moderation)
- Other Condiments: Fresh lemon juice, apple cider vinegar (if tolerated in small amounts)

Beverages:

- Herbal Teas: Chamomile, peppermint, ginger
- Water: Ensure you drink plenty of fresh, filtered water

Storage Essentials:

- Glass Containers: For storing leftovers and prepped ingredients to maintain freshness
- BPA-Free Plastic Containers: For pantry storage of dry goods
- Freezer Bags: For storing frozen fruits and vegetables

Pantry Tips:

- Rotate Stock: Regularly check and rotate your pantry items to ensure freshness and prevent histamine buildup in older foods.
- Labeling: Label containers with purchase dates to track freshness.

3.2 Must-Have Utensils and Appliances

Equipping your kitchen with the right utensils and appliances is essential for efficiently preparing and cooking low-histamine, vegetarian meals. Here's a comprehensive guide to the must-have tools that will make your kitchen functional and your cooking experience enjoyable:

1. Essential Utensils:

Chef's Knife:

A high-quality chef's knife is indispensable for chopping vegetables, fruits, and herbs. It ensures precision and safety in the kitchen.

Paring Knife:

A smaller knife is useful for peeling and slicing smaller fruits and vegetables.

Cutting Boards:

Have multiple cutting boards to avoid cross-contamination, preferably with separate boards for fruits, vegetables, and nuts.

Vegetable Peeler:

Essential for peeling root vegetables like carrots, sweet potatoes, and beets.

Grater/Zester:

Useful for grating fresh ginger, turmeric, and citrus zest.

Measuring Cups and Spoons:

Accurate measurements are crucial for following recipes and ensuring nutritional balance.

Mixing Bowls:

A set of various-sized mixing bowls is necessary for preparing ingredients and mixing salads, batters, and doughs.

Wooden Spoons and Spatulas:

Gentle on cookware, these are ideal for stirring, mixing, and sautéing.

Whisk:

For mixing dressings, batters, and sauces smoothly.

Tongs:

Handy for flipping and serving food, particularly when grilling or roasting vegetables.

Colander:

Essential for rinsing grains, legumes, and vegetables.

Sieve:

Useful for straining sauces and soups, or sifting dry ingredients.

Can Opener:

A sturdy can opener for opening canned beans and other preserved items.

Garlic Press:

For easily mincing garlic, a common ingredient in many low-histamine recipes.

Kitchen Shears:

Useful for snipping herbs, opening packages, and other miscellaneous tasks.

2. Essential Appliances:

High-Speed Blender:

Ideal for making smoothies, soups, sauces, and nut butters. It ensures smooth, consistent textures and blends ingredients thoroughly.

Food Processor:

Great for chopping vegetables, making dips, and processing nuts and seeds into flours or pastes.

Immersion Blender:

Convenient for blending soups and sauces directly in the pot without transferring hot liquids.

Rice Cooker:

Cook rice and other grains perfectly with minimal effort, freeing up stovetop space.

Slow Cooker:

Useful for preparing soups, stews, and legumes. However, be cautious as slow cooking can sometimes increase histamine levels in food.

Steamer Basket:

Fits into pots and allows you to steam vegetables, preserving nutrients and maintaining low histamine levels.

Instant Pot:

A versatile appliance that combines functions of a pressure cooker, slow cooker, rice cooker, and more. It's particularly useful for quickly cooking legumes and grains.

Toaster Oven:

Useful for small batch baking, roasting, and toasting without heating up the whole kitchen.

Electric Kettle:

Boil water quickly for teas, soups, and pre-soaking grains and legumes.

Dehydrator:

For drying fruits and vegetables, making low-histamine snacks, and preserving herbs.

3. Additional Useful Tools:

Mandoline Slicer:

For thinly slicing vegetables quickly and uniformly.

Spiralizer:

For making vegetable noodles, a great low-histamine and low-carb alternative to pasta.

Mortar and Pestle:

Useful for grinding fresh herbs and spices, creating pastes, and controlling texture.

Salad Spinner:

Ensures greens are thoroughly dried after washing, making them crisp and ready for salads.

Silicone Baking Mats:

Non-stick mats for baking without added fats or oils, making clean-up easier.

Glass Storage Containers:

For storing prepped ingredients and leftovers, maintaining freshness and reducing histamine build-up.

Mason Jars:

Versatile for storing dry goods, making overnight oats, or keeping homemade dressings and sauces.

Grill Pan:

For indoor grilling of vegetables and plant-based proteins, adding a charred flavor without outdoor equipment.

3.3 Tips for Meal Planning and Preparation

Effective meal planning and preparation are key to managing histamine intolerance on a vegetarian diet. With thoughtful planning, you can ensure that your meals are both nutritious and low in histamine. Here are some tips to help you plan and prepare your meals efficiently:

1. Meal Planning:

Create a Weekly Menu:

Plan your meals for the week in advance, including breakfast, lunch, dinner, and snacks. This helps ensure you have all the necessary ingredients and can reduce the likelihood of consuming high-histamine foods.

Focus on Fresh Ingredients:

Prioritize fresh, minimally processed vegetables, fruits, legumes, and grains. Fresh ingredients tend to have lower histamine levels compared to aged or processed foods.

Incorporate Variety:

Include a variety of low-histamine foods in your meal plan to ensure you get a wide range of nutrients. Rotate different vegetables, fruits, and protein sources throughout the week.

Batch Cooking:

Prepare larger quantities of meals that can be easily reheated or repurposed. For example, cook a big batch of lentils or quinoa and use them in different dishes throughout the week.

Balanced Meals:

Guarantee every dinner incorporates an equilibrium of protein, sound fats, and complex sugars. This keeps up with consistent energy levels and supports in general wellbeing.

2. Grocery Shopping:

Make a Shopping List:

Based on your weekly menu, create a detailed shopping list. This ensures you purchase only what you need and helps you avoid impulse buys of high-histamine or processed foods.

Shop Fresh and Local:

Whenever possible, buy fresh produce from local farmers' markets or grocery stores that restock frequently. This reduces the risk of consuming aged produce with higher histamine levels.

Check Labels:

When buying packaged foods, read labels carefully to avoid additives, preservatives, and other ingredients that can increase histamine levels.

3. Meal Preparation:

Prep Fresh Ingredients:

Wash, chop, and store fresh vegetables and fruits immediately after shopping. Use airtight containers to maintain freshness and prevent histamine buildup.

Use Appropriate Cooking Methods:

Opt for cooking methods that preserve nutrients and keep histamine levels low, such as steaming, boiling, and sautéing. Avoid slow-cooking or fermenting, as these methods can increase histamine levels.

Cook in Batches:

Prepare large batches of staple foods like grains, legumes, and soups. Portion them into individual servings and store them in the refrigerator or freezer for easy access throughout the week.

Plan for Leftovers:

Intentionally cook extra portions of meals that reheat well. This saves time and ensures you always have a low-histamine option available.

Label and Date:

Label and date all prepped and cooked foods before storing them. This helps you keep track of freshness and ensures you consume foods before they start to accumulate histamine.

4. Storing and Reheating:

Use Airtight Containers:

Store prepped ingredients and cooked meals in airtight glass or BPA-free plastic containers to maintain freshness and reduce histamine buildup.

Refrigerate Promptly:

Store leftovers in the refrigerator within two hours of cooking to prevent histamine formation. Consume refrigerated leftovers within 24-48 hours.

Freeze for Later:

Freeze portions of meals that you won't consume within a couple of days. Frozen foods can maintain their low-histamine levels if stored properly.

Reheat Safely:

Reheat food thoroughly but avoid reheating multiple times. Each time food is reheated, histamine levels can increase.

5. Smart Substitutions:

Replace High-Histamine Foods:

Substitute high-histamine ingredients with low-histamine alternatives. For example, use fresh herbs like basil and cilantro instead of aged spices, and opt for fresh vegetables over canned or fermented ones.

Experiment with New Recipes:

Explore new low-histamine vegetarian recipes to keep your meals interesting and diverse. Look for inspiration in cookbooks, online resources, and from other individuals managing histamine intolerance.

6. Staying Organized:

Keep a Food Diary:

Track what you eat and any side effects you experience. This helps identify potential triggers and refine your meal planning to better manage histamine intolerance.

Organize Your Kitchen:

Keep your kitchen organized and clutter-free. Store similar items together and make frequently used ingredients easily accessible to streamline meal preparation.

Plan for Busy Days:

Have quick, low-histamine meal options available for busy days when you don't have time to cook. This could include pre-made salads, smoothie packs, or simple grain and vegetable bowls.

Part II: Breakfasts to Energize Your Day

4. Refreshing Smoothies and Juices

4.1 Green Detox Smoothie

Ingredients:

- 1 cup fresh spinach
- 1/2 cup kale, stems removed
- 1/2 cucumber, chopped
- 1 green apple, cored and chopped
- 1/2 avocado
- 1 tablespoon chia seeds
- 1 tablespoon fresh lemon juice
- 1 teaspoon grated fresh ginger
- 1 cup coconut water or filtered water
- Optional: a few ice cubes for a colder smoothie

Directions:

1. Prepare Ingredients: Wash the spinach, kale, cucumber, and green apple thoroughly. Remove the stems from the kale and core the apple. Chop the cucumber and apple into smaller pieces for easier blending.
2. Blend Greens First: Add the spinach, kale, and cucumber to the blender. Pour in the coconut water or filtered water. Blend until the greens are fully broken down and smooth.
3. Add Remaining Ingredients: Add the chopped apple, avocado, chia seeds, lemon juice, and grated ginger to the blender. Blend again until smooth and creamy. If desired, add a few ice cubes and blend until they are crushed and incorporated.

4. Serve Immediately: Pour the smoothie into a glass and serve immediately to enjoy the fresh flavors and maximum nutrient content.

Serving Size:

Serves 1

Nutritional Information (per serving):

Calories: 220

Protein: 4g

Carbohydrates: 30g

Dietary Fiber: 11g

Sugars: 12g

Fat: 11g

Saturated Fat: 1.5g

Vitamin A: 150% DV

Vitamin C: 70% DV

Calcium: 10% DV

Iron: 15% DV

4.2 Berry Bliss Juice

Ingredients:

- 1 cup fresh blueberries
- 1 cup fresh raspberries
- 1 cup fresh strawberries, hulled
- 1/2 cup fresh blackberries
- 1 apple, cored and chopped
- 1/2 cucumber, chopped
- 1 tablespoon fresh lemon juice
- 1 cup filtered water
- Optional: a few ice cubes for a colder juice

Directions:

1. Prepare Ingredients: Wash all the berries, apple, and cucumber thoroughly. Hull the strawberries and core the apple. Chop the apple and cucumber into smaller pieces for easier blending.
2. Blend Fruits and Veggies: Add the blueberries, raspberries, strawberries, blackberries, apple, cucumber, and filtered water to the blender. Blend until the mixture is smooth.
3. Strain the Juice (Optional): For a smoother juice, strain the mixture through a fine mesh sieve or cheesecloth into a large bowl or pitcher. Use a spoon to press the pulp and extract as much juice as possible.
4. Add Lemon Juice: Stir in the fresh lemon juice to the strained juice.
5. Serve Immediately: Pour the Berry Bliss Juice into a glass and serve immediately. If desired, add a few ice cubes for a colder beverage.

Serving Size:

Serves 2

Nutritional Information (per serving):

Calories: 130

Protein: 2g

Carbohydrates: 32g

Dietary Fiber: 8g

Sugars: 21g

Fat: 1g

Saturated Fat: 0g

Vitamin A: 4% DV

Vitamin C: 120% DV

Calcium: 6% DV

Iron: 6% DV

4.3 Tropical Mango Smoothie

Ingredients:

- 1 ripe mango, peeled and chopped
- 1/2 cup pineapple chunks (fresh or frozen)
- 1/2 banana
- 1/2 cup coconut milk (unsweetened)
- 1/2 cup orange juice (freshly squeezed)
- 1 tablespoon chia seeds
- 1 teaspoon fresh lime juice
- Optional: a few ice cubes for a colder smoothie

Directions:

1. Prepare Ingredients: Peel and chop the mango and banana. If using fresh pineapple, chop it into chunks.
2. Blend Ingredients: Add the mango, pineapple, banana, coconut milk, orange juice, chia seeds, and lime juice to the blender. Blend until smooth and creamy. If desired, add a few ice cubes and blend until they are crushed and incorporated.
3. Serve Immediately: Pour the Tropical Mango Smoothie into a glass and serve immediately to enjoy the fresh flavors and maximum nutrient content.

Serving Size:

Serves 1

Nutritional Information (per serving):

Calories: 260
Protein: 3g
Carbohydrates: 50g
Dietary Fiber: 7g

Sugars: 35g

Fat: 9g

Saturated Fat: 7g

Vitamin A: 35% DV

Vitamin C: 160% DV

Calcium: 6% DV

Iron: 10% DV

4.4 Spinach and Pear Juice

Ingredients:

- 2 cups fresh spinach leaves
- 2 ripe pears, cored and chopped
- 1 cucumber, chopped
- 1/2 lemon, juiced
- 1/2 cup filtered water
- Optional: a few ice cubes for a colder juice

Directions:

1. Prepare Ingredients: Wash the spinach, pears, and cucumber thoroughly. Core and chop the pears. Chop the cucumber into smaller pieces.
2. Blend Ingredients: Add the spinach, pears, cucumber, lemon juice, and filtered water to the blender. Blend until smooth.
3. Strain the Juice (Optional): For a smoother juice, strain the mixture through a fine mesh sieve or cheesecloth into a large bowl or pitcher. Use a spoon to press the pulp and extract as much juice as possible.
4. Serve Immediately: Pour the Spinach and Pear Juice into a glass and serve immediately. If desired, add a few ice cubes for a colder beverage.

Serving Size:

Serves 2

Nutritional Information (per serving):

Calories: 90
Protein: 2g
Carbohydrates: 22g
Dietary Fiber: 4g

Sugars: 14g

Fat: 0.5g

Saturated Fat: 0g

Vitamin A: 50% DV

Vitamin C: 45% DV

Calcium: 6% DV

Iron: 8% DV

4.5 Watermelon Mint Smoothie

Ingredients:

- 2 cups watermelon, cubed and seeds removed
- 1/2 cucumber, chopped
- 1/2 cup coconut water (unsweetened)
- 1 tablespoon fresh mint leaves
- 1 teaspoon fresh lime juice
- Optional: a few ice cubes for a colder smoothie

Directions:

1. Prepare Ingredients: Cube the watermelon and remove any seeds. Chop the cucumber. Wash the mint leaves.
2. Blend Ingredients: Add the watermelon, cucumber, coconut water, mint leaves, and lime juice to the blender. Blend until smooth and well combined. If desired, add a few ice cubes and blend until they are crushed and incorporated.
3. Serve Immediately: Pour the Watermelon Mint Smoothie into a glass and serve immediately to enjoy the refreshing flavors and maximum nutrient content.

Serving Size:

Serves 2

Nutritional Information (per serving):

Calories: 60
Protein: 1g
Carbohydrates: 15g
Dietary Fiber: 1g
Sugars: 12g
Fat: 0.5g

Saturated Fat: 0g

Vitamin A: 10% DV

Vitamin C: 20% DV

Calcium: 2% DV

Iron: 2% DV

5. Hearty and Wholesome Breakfast Ideas

5.1 Quinoa Porridge with Fresh Berries

Ingredients:

- 1 cup quinoa, rinsed
- 2 cups almond milk (unsweetened) or other plant-based milk
- 1 tablespoon maple syrup (optional)
- 1 teaspoon vanilla extract
- 1/2 teaspoon ground cinnamon
- 1/2 cup fresh blueberries
- 1/2 cup fresh raspberries
- 1/2 cup fresh strawberries, hulled and sliced
- 1 tablespoon chia seeds
- 1 tablespoon almond slices (optional)

Directions:

1. Prepare Quinoa: Rinse the quinoa thoroughly under cold water to remove any bitterness.
2. Cook Quinoa: In a medium saucepan, combine the rinsed quinoa and almond milk. Bring to a boil over medium-high heat. Reduce the heat to low, cover, and simmer for about 15-20 minutes, or until the quinoa is tender and most of the liquid is absorbed.
3. Add Flavorings: Stir in the maple syrup (if using), vanilla extract, and ground cinnamon. Mix well.
4. Serve Porridge: Divide the quinoa porridge into bowls. Top each serving with fresh blueberries, raspberries, sliced strawberries, chia seeds, and almond slices (if using).

5. Serve Immediately: Enjoy the porridge warm for a nutritious and delicious breakfast.

Cooking Time:

Prep Time: 5 minutes

Cook Time: 20 minutes

Total Time: 25 minutes

Serving Size:

Serves 2

Nutritional Information (per serving):

Calories: 320

Protein: 9g

Carbohydrates: 56g

Dietary Fiber: 10g

Sugars: 14g

Fat: 8g

Saturated Fat: 1g

Vitamin A: 2% DV

Vitamin C: 50% DV

Calcium: 30% DV

Iron: 20% DV

5.2 Sweet Potato and Spinach Frittata

Ingredients:

- 1 large sweet potato, peeled and diced
- 1 tablespoon olive oil
- 1 small onion, finely chopped
- 2 cloves garlic, minced
- 3 cups fresh spinach leaves
- 6 large eggs
- 1/4 cup unsweetened almond milk or other plant-based milk
- 1/2 teaspoon salt
- 1/4 teaspoon black pepper
- 1/4 teaspoon smoked paprika (optional)
- 1 tablespoon fresh parsley, chopped (optional)

Directions:

1. Preheat Oven: Preheat your oven to 375°F (190°C).
2. Cook Sweet Potato: In a medium skillet, heat the olive oil over medium heat. Add the diced sweet potato and cook for about 10 minutes, stirring occasionally, until tender and slightly caramelized.
3. Add Onion and Garlic: Add the chopped onion to the skillet and cook for another 5 minutes, until softened. Stir in the minced garlic and cook for an additional 1 minute.
4. Wilt Spinach: Add the fresh spinach to the skillet and cook until wilted, about 2-3 minutes. Remove the skillet from heat and set aside.
5. Prepare Egg Mixture: In a large bowl, whisk together the eggs, almond milk, salt, black pepper, and smoked paprika (if using).
6. Combine Ingredients: Add the cooked sweet potato, onion, garlic, and spinach mixture to the bowl with the eggs. Stir to combine evenly.

7. Bake Frittata: Pour the mixture into a greased 9-inch pie dish or oven-safe skillet. Bake in the preheated oven for 20-25 minutes, or until the frittata is set and a knife inserted in the center comes out clean.

8. Serve: Let the frittata cool for a few minutes before slicing. Garnish with fresh parsley if desired.

Serving Size:

Serves 4

Nutritional Information (per serving):

Calories: 180

Protein: 9g

Carbohydrates: 16g

Dietary Fiber: 3g

Sugars: 4g

Fat: 9g

Saturated Fat: 2g

Vitamin A: 210% DV

Vitamin C: 20% DV

Calcium: 10% DV

Iron: 15% DV

5.3 Avocado Toast with Radishes

Ingredients:

- 2 ripe avocados
- 1 tablespoon fresh lemon juice
- 1/2 teaspoon salt
- 1/4 teaspoon black pepper
- 4 slices whole-grain bread (gluten-free if preferred)
- 6 radishes, thinly sliced
- 1 tablespoon fresh chives, chopped
- 1 tablespoon extra-virgin olive oil
- Optional: pinch of red pepper flakes for garnish

Directions:

1. Prepare Avocado Mixture: Cut the avocados in half, remove the pits, and scoop the flesh into a bowl. Add the lemon juice, salt, and black pepper. Mash the avocado mixture with a fork until it reaches your desired consistency (smooth or slightly chunky).
2. Toast Bread: While preparing the avocado mixture, toast the slices of whole-grain bread until they are golden brown and crisp.
3. Assemble Avocado Toast: Spread the mashed avocado mixture evenly onto each slice of toasted bread.
4. Add Toppings: Arrange the thinly sliced radishes on top of the avocado spread. Sprinkle with chopped chives and drizzle with extra-virgin olive oil. If desired, add a pinch of red pepper flakes for a bit of heat.
5. Serve Immediately: Serve the avocado toast immediately to enjoy the fresh flavors and textures.

Cooking Time:

Prep Time: 10 minutes
Total Time: 10 minutes
Serving Size:

Serves 2 (2 slices each)
Nutritional Information (per serving):

Calories: 360
Protein: 6g
Carbohydrates: 38g
Dietary Fiber: 13g
Sugars: 2g
Fat: 23g
Saturated Fat: 3g
Vitamin A: 6% DV
Vitamin C: 25% DV
Calcium: 8% DV
Iron: 15% DV

5.4 Chia Seed Pudding with Almond Milk

Ingredients:

- 1/4 cup chia seeds
- 1 cup unsweetened almond milk (or other plant-based milk)
- 1 tablespoon maple syrup (optional)
- 1/2 teaspoon vanilla extract
- Fresh fruit for topping (e.g., berries, sliced banana, kiwi)
- Nuts or seeds for topping (e.g., almonds, pumpkin seeds)

Directions:

1. Mix Ingredients: In a medium bowl, combine the chia seeds, almond milk, maple syrup (if using), and vanilla extract. Stir well to ensure the chia seeds are evenly distributed.
2. Refrigerate: Cover the bowl and refrigerate for at least 4 hours or overnight. Stir the mixture after the first hour to prevent clumping.
3. Serve: Once the pudding has thickened to a gel-like consistency, give it a good stir. Divide the chia seed pudding into serving bowls.
4. Add Toppings: Top with fresh fruit and a sprinkle of nuts or seeds. Serve immediately.

Cooking Time:

Prep Time: 5 minutes

Chill Time: 4 hours (or overnight)

Total Time: 4 hours and 5 minutes

Serving Size:

Serves 2

Nutritional Information (per serving):

Calories: 180

Protein: 5g

Carbohydrates: 19g

Dietary Fiber: 11g

Sugars: 4g

Fat: 9g

Saturated Fat: 1g

Vitamin A: 2% DV

Vitamin C: 10% DV

Calcium: 35% DV

Iron: 15% DV

5.5 Buckwheat Pancakes with Maple Syrup

Ingredients:

- 1 cup buckwheat flour
- 1 tablespoon baking powder
- 1/2 teaspoon salt
- 1 tablespoon maple syrup (plus more for serving)
- 1 cup unsweetened almond milk (or other plant-based milk)
- 1 teaspoon vanilla extract
- 2 tablespoons coconut oil, melted (plus more for cooking)
- Fresh fruit for topping (e.g., blueberries, sliced strawberries)

Directions:

1. Mix Dry Ingredients: In a large bowl, whisk together the buckwheat flour, baking powder, and salt.
2. Mix Wet Ingredients: In another bowl, combine the almond milk, maple syrup, vanilla extract, and melted coconut oil. Mix well.
3. Combine Wet and Dry Ingredients: Pour the wet ingredients into the dry ingredients and stir until just combined. Be careful not to overmix; a few lumps are fine.
4. Preheat Pan: Heat a non-stick skillet or griddle over medium heat and lightly grease with a small amount of coconut oil.
5. Cook Pancakes: Pour 1/4 cup of batter onto the skillet for each pancake. Cook for 2-3 minutes, or until bubbles form on the surface and the edges look set. Flip and cook for another 2-3 minutes, or until golden brown and cooked through.
6. Serve: Serve the pancakes warm, topped with fresh fruit and a drizzle of maple syrup.

Cooking Time:

Prep Time: 10 minutes

Cook Time: 20 minutes

Total Time: 30 minutes

Serving Size:

Serves 2 (makes about 8 pancakes)

Nutritional Information (per serving):

Calories: 340

Protein: 6g

Carbohydrates: 55g

Dietary Fiber: 6g

Sugars: 12g

Fat: 12g

Saturated Fat: 7g

Vitamin A: 0% DV

Vitamin C: 0% DV

Calcium: 30% DV

Iron: 15% DV

Part III: Satisfying Lunches and Light Bites

6. Creative Salads and Dressings

6.1 Zucchini Noodle Salad with Lemon-Tahini Dressing

Ingredients:

For the Salad:

- 3 medium zucchinis, spiralized into noodles
- 1 cup cherry tomatoes, halved
- 1/2 red bell pepper, thinly sliced
- 1/2 cucumber, thinly sliced
- 1/4 red onion, thinly sliced
- 1/4 cup fresh parsley, chopped

For the Lemon-Tahini Dressing:

- 1/4 cup tahini
- 2 tablespoons fresh lemon juice
- 1 tablespoon olive oil
- 1 tablespoon maple syrup (optional)
- 1 clove garlic, minced
- 1/4 teaspoon salt
- 1/4 teaspoon black pepper
- 2-4 tablespoons water (to thin, as needed)

Directions:

1. Prepare Zucchini Noodles: Using a spiralizer, create noodles from the zucchinis. Place the zucchini noodles in a large salad bowl.

2. Prepare Vegetables: Add the cherry tomatoes, red bell pepper, cucumber, red onion, and chopped parsley to the bowl with the zucchini noodles.

3. Make the Dressing: In a small bowl, whisk together the tahini, lemon juice, olive oil, maple syrup (if using), minced garlic, salt, and black pepper. Add water a tablespoon at a time until the dressing reaches your desired consistency (creamy but pourable).

4. Toss the Salad: Pour the lemon-tahini dressing over the salad and toss gently to combine, ensuring all the vegetables are coated with the dressing.

5. Serve Immediately: Serve the Zucchini Noodle Salad fresh. It can also be chilled for 10-15 minutes if a colder salad is preferred.

Serving Size:

Serves 4

Nutritional Information (per serving):

Calories: 180

Protein: 5g

Carbohydrates: 16g

Dietary Fiber: 5g

Sugars: 7g

Fat: 12g

Saturated Fat: 2g

Vitamin A: 20% DV

Vitamin C: 70% DV

Calcium: 8% DV

Iron: 10% DV

6.2 Lentil and Roasted Vegetable Salad

Ingredients:

For the Salad:

- 1 cup green or brown lentils, rinsed
- 2 cups water or vegetable broth
- 1 red bell pepper, chopped
- 1 yellow bell pepper, chopped
- 1 small eggplant, diced
- 1 zucchini, diced
- 1 red onion, chopped
- 2 tablespoons olive oil
- 1 teaspoon salt
- 1/2 teaspoon black pepper
- 1 teaspoon dried thyme
- 1 teaspoon dried oregano
- 1/4 cup fresh parsley, chopped

For the Dressing:

- 3 tablespoons olive oil
- 2 tablespoons fresh lemon juice
- 1 tablespoon apple cider vinegar
- 1 teaspoon Dijon mustard (optional)
- 1 clove garlic, minced
- Salt and pepper to taste

Directions:

1. Cook Lentils: In a medium saucepan, combine the lentils and water or vegetable broth. Bring to a boil, then reduce heat and simmer for 20-25 minutes, or until lentils are tender but not mushy. Drain and set aside to cool.

2. Preheat Oven: Preheat your oven to 400°F (200°C).

3. Prepare Vegetables: On a large baking sheet, toss the red bell pepper, yellow bell pepper, eggplant, zucchini, and red onion with 2 tablespoons of olive oil, salt, black pepper, thyme, and oregano. Spread the vegetables out in an even layer.

4. Roast Vegetables: Roast the vegetables in the preheated oven for 20-25 minutes, or until they are tender and slightly caramelized. Remove from the oven and let cool slightly.

5. Make Dressing: In a small bowl, whisk together the olive oil, lemon juice, apple cider vinegar, Dijon mustard (if using), minced garlic, salt, and pepper until well combined.

6. Assemble Salad: In a large bowl, combine the cooked lentils, roasted vegetables, and chopped parsley. Drizzle the dressing over the salad and toss gently to combine.

7. Serve: Serve the salad warm or at room temperature.

Cooking Time:

Prep Time: 15 minutes
Cook Time: 25 minutes

Total Time: 40 minutes

Serving Size:

Serves 4

Nutritional Information (per serving):

Calories: 300

Protein: 10g

Carbohydrates: 40g

Dietary Fiber: 15g

Sugars: 8g

Fat: 12g

Saturated Fat: 2g

Vitamin A: 25% DV

Vitamin C: 120% DV

Calcium: 6% DV

Iron: 25% DV

6.3 Greek Salad with Feta and Olives

Ingredients:

For the Salad:

- 3 cups chopped Romaine lettuce
- 1 cup cherry tomatoes, halved
- 1 cucumber, diced
- 1/2 red onion, thinly sliced
- 1 green bell pepper, chopped
- 1/2 cup Kalamata olives, pitted and halved
- 1/2 cup feta cheese, crumbled
- 2 tablespoons fresh parsley, chopped

For the Dressing:

- 1/4 cup extra-virgin olive oil
- 2 tablespoons red wine vinegar
- 1 teaspoon dried oregano
- 1 clove garlic, minced
- Salt and pepper to taste

Directions:

1. Prepare Vegetables: In a large salad bowl, combine the chopped Romaine lettuce, cherry tomatoes, cucumber, red onion, and green bell pepper.
2. Add Olives and Feta: Add the Kalamata olives and crumbled feta cheese to the bowl. Toss gently to combine.
3. Make Dressing: In a small bowl, whisk together the olive oil, red wine vinegar, dried oregano, minced garlic, salt, and pepper until well combined.

4. Dress the Salad: Pour the dressing over the salad and toss gently to ensure all the ingredients are well coated.

5. Garnish and Serve: Garnish with chopped parsley and serve immediately.

Cooking Time:

Prep Time: 15 minutes

Total Time: 15 minutes

Serving Size:

Serves 4

Nutritional Information (per serving):

Calories: 250

Protein: 6g

Carbohydrates: 10g

Dietary Fiber: 3g

Sugars: 4g

Fat: 22g

Saturated Fat: 6g

Vitamin A: 45% DV

Vitamin C: 70% DV

Calcium: 15% DV

Iron: 10% DV

6.4 Roasted Beet and Arugula Salad

Ingredients:

For the Salad:

- 4 medium beets, scrubbed and trimmed
- 4 cups arugula
- 1/4 red onion, thinly sliced
- 1/2 cup walnuts, toasted
- 1/4 cup crumbled goat cheese (optional)
- 1 tablespoon fresh chives, chopped

For the Dressing:

- 3 tablespoons extra-virgin olive oil
- 2 tablespoons balsamic vinegar
- 1 teaspoon Dijon mustard (optional)
- 1 teaspoon maple syrup (optional)
- Salt and pepper to taste

Directions:

1. Roast Beets: Preheat your oven to 400°F (200°C). Wrap each beet individually in aluminum foil and place them on a baking sheet. Roast for 45-60 minutes, or until the beets are tender when pierced with a fork. Allow the beets to cool, then peel and cut into wedges or slices.
2. Prepare Salad Base: While the beets are roasting, place the arugula in a large salad bowl. Add the thinly sliced red onion.
3. Toast Walnuts: In a dry skillet over medium heat, toast the walnuts for 5-7 minutes, stirring frequently, until fragrant and lightly browned. Remove from heat and let cool.

4. Make Dressing: In a small bowl, whisk together the olive oil, balsamic vinegar, Dijon mustard (if using), maple syrup (if using), salt, and pepper until well combined.
5. Assemble Salad: Add the roasted beets and toasted walnuts to the salad bowl with the arugula and red onion. Drizzle the dressing over the salad and toss gently to combine.
6. Add Toppings: Sprinkle the salad with crumbled goat cheese (if using) and chopped chives.
7. Serve Immediately: Serve the salad fresh. It can also be chilled for a few minutes if a colder salad is preferred.

Cooking Time:

Prep Time: 15 minutes
Cook Time: 45-60 minutes (roasting beets)
Total Time: 1 hour 15 minutes

Serving Size:

Serves 4

Nutritional Information (per serving):

Calories: 250
Protein: 5g
Carbohydrates: 18g
Dietary Fiber: 5g
Sugars: 10g
Fat: 18g
Saturated Fat: 3g
Vitamin A: 15% DV
Vitamin C: 20% DV
Calcium: 8% DV

Iron: 10% DV

6.5 Quinoa and Black Bean Salad with Lime Dressing

Ingredients:

For the Salad:

- 1 cup quinoa, rinsed
- 2 cups water
- 1 can (15 oz) black beans, rinsed and drained
- 1 red bell pepper, chopped
- 1 cup corn kernels (fresh or frozen)
- 1/2 red onion, finely chopped
- 1 avocado, diced
- 1/4 cup fresh cilantro, chopped

For the Lime Dressing:

- 1/4 cup extra-virgin olive oil
- 3 tablespoons fresh lime juice
- 1 clove garlic, minced
- 1 teaspoon ground cumin
- 1 teaspoon maple syrup (optional)
- Salt and pepper to taste

Directions:

1. Cook Quinoa: In a medium saucepan, bring the water to a boil. Add the quinoa, reduce the heat to low, cover, and simmer for 15 minutes or until the water is absorbed and the quinoa is tender. Remove from heat and let it sit, covered, for 5 minutes. Fluff with a fork and let it cool.

2. Prepare Vegetables: While the quinoa is cooking, chop the red bell pepper, dice the red onion, and prepare the other vegetables.

3. Combine Salad Ingredients: In a large bowl, combine the cooked quinoa, black beans, red bell pepper, corn, red onion, avocado, and fresh cilantro.

4. Make Dressing: In a small bowl, whisk together the olive oil, fresh lime juice, minced garlic, ground cumin, maple syrup (if using), salt, and pepper until well combined.

5. Dress the Salad: Pour the lime dressing over the quinoa and vegetable mixture. Toss gently to combine, ensuring all the ingredients are well coated with the dressing.

6. Serve Immediately: Serve the salad fresh, or chill it in the refrigerator for 15-20 minutes if a colder salad is preferred.

Cooking Time:

Prep Time: 15 minutes
Cook Time: 20 minutes
Total Time: 35 minutes
Serving Size:

Serves 4
Nutritional Information (per serving):

Calories: 320
Protein: 8g
Carbohydrates: 38g

Dietary Fiber: 10g

Sugars: 5g

Fat: 16g

Saturated Fat: 2g

Vitamin A: 25% DV

Vitamin C: 60% DV

Calcium: 6% DV

Iron: 15% DV

7. Delicious Wraps and Sandwiches

7.1 Chickpea and Avocado Wrap

Ingredients:

For the Wrap Filling:

- 1 can (15 oz) chickpeas, rinsed and drained
- 1 ripe avocado
- 1 tablespoon fresh lemon juice
- 1 tablespoon extra-virgin olive oil
- 1 clove garlic, minced
- 1/4 teaspoon salt
- 1/4 teaspoon black pepper
- 1/2 teaspoon ground cumin
- 1/4 teaspoon paprika
- 1/4 cup red onion, finely chopped
- 1/4 cup fresh cilantro, chopped
- 2 large whole wheat or gluten-free tortillas
- 1 cup fresh spinach leaves
- 1/2 cup cherry tomatoes, halved
- 1/4 cup shredded carrots

Directions:

1. Prepare Chickpea Mixture: In a large bowl, mash the chickpeas and avocado together using a fork or potato masher until well combined but still slightly chunky.
2. Add Seasonings: Stir in the fresh lemon juice, olive oil, minced garlic, salt, black pepper, ground cumin, and paprika. Mix until well combined.

3. Add Vegetables: Fold in the red onion and fresh cilantro until evenly distributed.

4. Assemble Wraps: Lay the tortillas flat and evenly divide the chickpea and avocado mixture between them, spreading it in the center of each tortilla.

5. Add Spinach and Toppings: Top the chickpea mixture with fresh spinach leaves, cherry tomatoes, and shredded carrots.

6. Wrap and Serve: Fold in the sides of the tortilla and then roll it up tightly from the bottom to create a wrap. Cut each wrap in half and serve immediately.

Cooking Time:

Prep Time: 15 minutes

Total Time: 15 minutes

Serving Size:

Serves 2

Nutritional Information (per serving):

Calories: 380

Protein: 11g

Carbohydrates: 48g

Dietary Fiber: 13g

Sugars: 6g

Fat: 17g

Saturated Fat: 2g

Vitamin A: 70% DV

Vitamin C: 35% DV

Calcium: 10% DV

Iron: 20% DV

7.2 Grilled Veggie and Hummus Sandwich

Ingredients:

For the Sandwich:

- 1 zucchini, sliced lengthwise
- 1 yellow squash, sliced lengthwise
- 1 red bell pepper, seeded and quartered
- 1/2 red onion, sliced into thick rings
- 4 slices whole grain bread or gluten-free bread
- 1/2 cup hummus
- 1 tablespoon olive oil
- Salt and pepper to taste
- Fresh spinach leaves (optional)
- 1/4 cup fresh basil leaves

Directions:

1. Prepare Vegetables: Preheat a grill pan or outdoor grill over medium-high heat. Brush the zucchini, yellow squash, red bell pepper, and red onion with olive oil and season with salt and pepper.

2. Grill Vegetables: Grill the vegetables for 3-4 minutes per side, or until tender and grill marks appear. Remove from heat and set aside.

3. Assemble Sandwiches:

- Spread hummus evenly on each slice of bread.
- Layer grilled zucchini, yellow squash, red bell pepper, and red onion on two slices of bread.

- Top with fresh spinach leaves (if using) and fresh basil leaves.
- Place the remaining slices of bread on top to close the sandwiches.

4. Grill Sandwiches: Heat a grill pan or skillet over medium heat. Place the sandwiches on the grill pan and cook for 2-3 minutes per side, or until the bread is toasted and golden brown.

5. Serve: Remove from heat and let cool slightly before slicing in half. Serve warm.

Cooking Time:

Prep Time: 15 minutes

Cook Time: 10 minutes

Total Time: 25 minutes

Serving Size:

Serves 2

Nutritional Information (per serving):

Calories: 350

Protein: 12g

Carbohydrates: 45g

Dietary Fiber: 10g

Sugars: 9g

Fat: 15g

Saturated Fat: 2g

Vitamin A: 40% DV

Vitamin C: 120% DV

Calcium: 15% DV

Iron: 20% DV

7.3 Tofu and Veggie Wrap with Peanut Sauce

Ingredients:

For the Wrap:

- 1 block (14 oz) firm tofu, drained and pressed
- 1 tablespoon soy sauce or tamari
- 1 tablespoon olive oil
- 1/2 teaspoon ground cumin
- 1/2 teaspoon paprika
- Salt and pepper to taste
- 2 large whole wheat or gluten-free tortillas
- 1 cup shredded red cabbage
- 1/2 cup shredded carrots
- 1/2 cup cucumber, julienned
- 1/4 cup fresh cilantro leaves

For the Peanut Sauce:

- 1/4 cup natural peanut butter
- 2 tablespoons soy sauce or tamari
- 2 tablespoons lime juice
- 1 tablespoon maple syrup or honey
- 1 clove garlic, minced
- 1/2 teaspoon grated fresh ginger
- Water, as needed to thin

Directions:

1. Prepare Tofu: Cut the pressed tofu into thin strips. In a bowl, combine the soy sauce or tamari, olive oil, ground cumin, paprika, salt, and pepper. Add the tofu strips and toss gently to coat.

2. Cook Tofu: Heat a skillet over medium-high heat. Add the tofu strips in a single layer and cook for 3-4 minutes per side, or until golden brown and crispy. Remove from heat and set aside.

3. Prepare Peanut Sauce: In a small bowl, whisk together the peanut butter, soy sauce or tamari, lime juice, maple syrup or honey, minced garlic, and grated fresh ginger. Add water, a tablespoon at a time, until desired consistency is reached.

4. Assemble Wraps:

- Lay the tortillas flat and spread a generous amount of peanut sauce on each.
- Divide the shredded red cabbage, shredded carrots, julienned cucumber, crispy tofu strips, and fresh cilantro leaves evenly between the tortillas.

5. Wrap and Serve: Fold in the sides of the tortilla and then roll it up tightly from the bottom to create a wrap. Cut each wrap in half and serve immediately.

Cooking Time:

Prep Time: 20 minutes
Cook Time: 10 minutes
Total Time: 30 minutes
Serving Size:

Serves 2

Nutritional Information (per serving):

Calories: 500
Protein: 27g
Carbohydrates: 45g
Dietary Fiber: 8g
Sugars: 11g
Fat: 27g
Saturated Fat: 5g
Vitamin A: 150% DV
Vitamin C: 40% DV
Calcium: 25% DV
Iron: 30% DV

7.4 Portobello Mushroom Burger

Ingredients:

For the Mushroom Burger:

- 4 large portobello mushroom caps, stems removed
- 2 tablespoons balsamic vinegar
- 2 tablespoons soy sauce or tamari
- 2 cloves garlic, minced
- 2 tablespoons olive oil
- Salt and pepper to taste
- 4 whole grain burger buns or lettuce wraps
- 1/2 cup hummus or vegan mayonnaise
- 1 cup fresh spinach leaves
- 1 large tomato, sliced
- 1/2 red onion, thinly sliced
- 1 avocado, sliced

Optional Toppings:

- Sliced pickles
- Mustard
- Sprouts

Directions:

1. Marinate Mushrooms: In a shallow dish, whisk together the balsamic vinegar, soy sauce or tamari, minced garlic, olive oil, salt, and pepper. Place the portobello mushroom caps in the marinade, turning to coat. Let them marinate for at least 15 minutes, flipping once.

2. Grill Mushrooms: Preheat a grill or grill pan over medium-high heat. Grill the marinated mushroom caps for 4-5 minutes per side, or until tender and grill marks appear.

3. Prepare Buns or Lettuce Wraps: While the mushrooms are grilling, lightly toast the whole grain burger buns on the grill or in a toaster. If using lettuce wraps, wash and dry large lettuce leaves.

4. Assemble Burgers:

- Spread a generous amount of hummus or vegan mayonnaise on the bottom half of each burger bun or lettuce wrap.
- Layer with fresh spinach leaves, grilled portobello mushroom caps, tomato slices, red onion slices, and avocado slices.
- Add any optional toppings, such as sliced pickles, mustard, or sprouts.

5. Serve Immediately: Place the top half of the burger bun or wrap on top. Serve immediately while warm.

Cooking Time:

Prep Time: 15 minutes
Cook Time: 10 minutes
Total Time: 25 minutes (plus marinating time)
Serving Size:

Serves 4
Nutritional Information (per serving):

Calories: 350
Protein: 10g

Carbohydrates: 40g

Dietary Fiber: 10g

Sugars: 7g

Fat: 18g

Saturated Fat: 3g

Vitamin A: 40% DV

Vitamin C: 25% DV

Calcium: 10% DV

Iron: 15% DV

7.5 Roasted Red Pepper and Spinach Panini

Ingredients:

For the Panini:

- 4 slices whole grain bread or gluten-free bread
- 1/2 cup roasted red peppers (from a jar), drained and sliced
- 1 cup fresh spinach leaves
- 1/4 cup sliced black olives (optional)
- 4 slices provolone cheese or vegan cheese
- 2 tablespoons olive oil or softened butter

Optional Seasonings:

- Dried oregano
- Garlic powder
- Red pepper flakes

Directions:

1. Prepare Panini Press or Skillet: Preheat a panini press or a large skillet over medium heat.

2. Assemble Panini:

- Lay out the slices of bread on a clean surface.
- On two slices of bread, layer roasted red peppers, fresh spinach leaves, sliced black olives (if using), and slices of provolone or vegan cheese.
- Sprinkle with optional seasonings like dried oregano, garlic powder, and red pepper flakes, if desired.
- Top each sandwich with the remaining slices of bread.

3. Grill Panini:

- Brush the outsides of the sandwiches with olive oil or spread with softened butter.
- Place the sandwiches in the preheated panini press or skillet.
- If using a skillet, place a heavy pan or a sandwich press on top of the sandwiches to press them down.

4. Cook Panini: Grill for 3-4 minutes per side, or until the bread is golden brown and the cheese is melted.

6. Serve: Remove from the panini press or skillet. Let cool slightly before slicing in half. Serve warm.

Cooking Time:

Prep Time: 10 minutes
Cook Time: 8 minutes
Total Time: 18 minutes
Serving Size:

Serves 2
Nutritional Information (per serving):

Calories: 400
Protein: 15g
Carbohydrates: 30g
Dietary Fiber: 5g
Sugars: 3g
Fat: 25g
Saturated Fat: 9g

Vitamin A: 60% DV
Vitamin C: 40% DV
Calcium: 30% DV
Iron: 15% DV

Part IV: Nutritious and Flavorful Dinners

8. Hearty Soups and Stews

8.1 Carrot and Ginger Soup

Ingredients:

- 2 tablespoons olive oil
- 1 large onion, chopped
- 3 cloves garlic, minced
- 1 tablespoon fresh ginger, minced
- 6 large carrots, peeled and chopped
- 4 cups vegetable broth (low-sodium)
- 1 cup coconut milk (optional for creaminess)
- 1 teaspoon ground cumin
- 1 teaspoon ground coriander
- Salt and pepper to taste
- Fresh cilantro or parsley for garnish

Directions:

1. Sauté Aromatics: In a large pot, heat the olive oil over medium heat. Add the chopped onion and cook until softened, about 5 minutes. Add the minced garlic and ginger, and cook for an additional 2 minutes, until fragrant.

2. Add Carrots and Spices: Add the chopped carrots, ground cumin, and ground coriander to the pot. Stir well to coat the carrots with the spices.

3. Simmer Soup: Pour in the vegetable broth and bring to a boil. Reduce heat to a simmer and cook until the carrots are tender, about 20 minutes.

4. Blend Soup: Use an immersion blender to puree the soup until smooth. Alternatively, carefully transfer the soup to a blender in batches and blend until smooth. If using a blender, return the soup to the pot.

5. Add Coconut Milk (optional): Stir in the coconut milk if you prefer a creamier soup. Heat through for an additional 5 minutes. Season with salt and pepper to taste.

6. Serve: Ladle the soup into bowls and garnish with fresh cilantro or parsley. Serve hot.

Cooking Time:

Prep Time: 10 minutes
Cook Time: 30 minutes
Total Time: 40 minutes
Serving Size:

Serves 4
Nutritional Information (per serving):

Calories: 200
Protein: 3g
Carbohydrates: 22g
Dietary Fiber: 5g
Sugars: 10g
Fat: 12g
Saturated Fat: 5g
Vitamin A: 450% DV

Vitamin C: 15% DV
Calcium: 6% DV
Iron: 8% DV

8.2 Butternut Squash Stew

Ingredients:

- 2 tablespoons olive oil
- 1 large onion, chopped
- 3 cloves garlic, minced
- 1 large butternut squash, peeled, seeded, and cubed
- 2 large carrots, peeled and chopped
- 2 stalks celery, chopped
- 1 large potato, peeled and cubed
- 4 cups vegetable broth (low-sodium)
- 1 can (14.5 oz) diced tomatoes (no salt added)
- 1 teaspoon ground cumin
- 1 teaspoon smoked paprika
- 1/2 teaspoon ground cinnamon
- 1/2 teaspoon ground turmeric
- Salt and pepper to taste
- 1/4 cup fresh parsley, chopped (for garnish)

Directions:

1. Sauté Aromatics: In a large pot, heat the olive oil over medium heat. Add the chopped onion and cook until softened, about 5 minutes. Add the minced garlic and cook for an additional 1-2 minutes until fragrant.

2. Add Vegetables and Spices: Add the cubed butternut squash, chopped carrots, chopped celery, and cubed potato to the pot. Stir well to combine. Add the ground cumin, smoked paprika, ground cinnamon, and ground turmeric. Stir to coat the vegetables with the spices.

3. Simmer Stew: Pour in the vegetable broth and diced tomatoes. Bring to a boil, then reduce the heat to a simmer. Cover and cook for about 30-35 minutes, or until the vegetables are tender.

4. Season and Serve: Taste and adjust seasoning with salt and pepper. Ladle the stew into bowls and garnish with fresh parsley. Serve hot.

Cooking Time:

Prep Time: 15 minutes

Cook Time: 35 minutes

Total Time: 50 minutes

Serving Size:

Serves 4

Nutritional Information (per serving):

Calories: 250

Protein: 4g

Carbohydrates: 50g

Dietary Fiber: 10g

Sugars: 12g

Fat: 6g

Saturated Fat: 1g

Vitamin A: 400% DV

Vitamin C: 50% DV

Calcium: 10% DV

Iron: 15% DV

8.3 Sweet Potato and Lentil Soup

Ingredients:

- 2 tablespoons olive oil
- 1 large onion, chopped
- 3 cloves garlic, minced
- 2 large sweet potatoes, peeled and cubed
- 1 cup red lentils, rinsed and drained
- 1 can (14.5 oz) diced tomatoes (no salt added)
- 4 cups vegetable broth (low-sodium)
- 1 teaspoon ground cumin
- 1 teaspoon ground coriander
- 1/2 teaspoon ground turmeric
- 1/2 teaspoon smoked paprika
- 1/4 teaspoon cayenne pepper (optional, for heat)
- Salt and pepper to taste
- 1/4 cup fresh cilantro or parsley, chopped (for garnish)
- 1 tablespoon lemon juice (optional, for added brightness)

Directions:

1. Sauté Aromatics: In a large pot, heat the olive oil over medium heat. Add the chopped onion and cook until softened, about 5 minutes. Add the minced garlic and cook for an additional 1-2 minutes, until fragrant.

2. Add Sweet Potatoes and Spices: Add the cubed sweet potatoes to the pot. Stir in the ground cumin, ground coriander, ground turmeric, smoked paprika, and cayenne pepper (if using). Cook for 2-3 minutes, stirring to coat the sweet potatoes with the spices.

3. Simmer Soup: Add the rinsed red lentils, diced tomatoes, and vegetable broth to the pot. Bring to a boil, then reduce the heat to a simmer. Cover and cook for about 25-30 minutes, or until the sweet potatoes and lentils are tender.

4. Blend (Optional): For a smoother soup, use an immersion blender to partially blend the soup until you reach the desired consistency. Alternatively, you can transfer half of the soup to a blender, blend until smooth, and then return it to the pot.

5. Season and Serve: Stir in the lemon juice (if using) and season with salt and pepper to taste. Ladle the soup into bowls and garnish with fresh cilantro or parsley. Serve hot.

Cooking Time:

Prep Time: 10 minutes
Cook Time: 30 minutes
Total Time: 40 minutes
Serving Size:

Serves 4
Nutritional Information (per serving):

Calories: 320
Protein: 10g
Carbohydrates: 55g
Dietary Fiber: 15g
Sugars: 10g
Fat: 8g
Saturated Fat: 1g

Vitamin A: 350% DV

Vitamin C: 35% DV

Calcium: 10% DV

Iron: 20% DV

8.4 Tomato Basil Soup (Low-Histamine)

Ingredients:

- 2 tablespoons olive oil
- 1 large onion, chopped
- 3 cloves garlic, minced
- 6 large fresh tomatoes, peeled and chopped (or 2 cans (14.5 oz) no-salt-added diced tomatoes)
- 2 cups vegetable broth (low-sodium)
- 1/4 cup fresh basil leaves, chopped
- 1 tablespoon tomato paste (optional, for deeper flavor)
- 1 teaspoon dried oregano
- Salt and pepper to taste
- 1/2 cup coconut milk (optional, for creaminess)
- Fresh basil leaves for garnish

Directions:

1. Sauté Aromatics: In a large pot, heat the olive oil over medium heat. Add the chopped onion and cook until softened, about 5 minutes. Add the minced garlic and cook for an additional 1-2 minutes until fragrant.

2. Add Tomatoes and Broth: Add the peeled and chopped fresh tomatoes (or canned diced tomatoes) to the pot. Stir in the vegetable broth.

3. Simmer Soup: Bring the mixture to a boil, then reduce the heat to a simmer. Cook for about 20 minutes, allowing the flavors to meld together.

4. Add Herbs and Seasoning: Stir in the chopped fresh basil leaves, dried oregano, and tomato paste (if using). Season with salt and pepper to taste. Simmer for an additional 5 minutes.

5. Blend Soup: Use an immersion blender to puree the soup until smooth. Alternatively, carefully transfer the soup to a blender in batches and blend until smooth. If using a blender, return the soup to the pot.

6. Add Coconut Milk (Optional): Stir in the coconut milk if you prefer a creamier soup. Heat through for an additional 5 minutes.

7. Serve: Ladle the soup into bowls and garnish with fresh basil leaves. Serve hot.

Cooking Time:

Prep Time: 10 minutes
Cook Time: 30 minutes
Total Time: 40 minutes
Serving Size:

Serves 4
Nutritional Information (per serving):

Calories: 180
Protein: 3g
Carbohydrates: 20g
Dietary Fiber: 5g
Sugars: 12g
Fat: 10g
Saturated Fat: 4g

Vitamin A: 30% DV

Vitamin C: 40% DV

Calcium: 8% DV

Iron: 10% DV

8.5 Chickpea and Spinach Stew

Ingredients:

- 2 tablespoons olive oil
- 1 large onion, chopped
- 3 cloves garlic, minced
- 1 teaspoon ground cumin
- 1 teaspoon ground coriander
- 1 teaspoon smoked paprika
- 1/2 teaspoon ground turmeric
- 1/4 teaspoon cayenne pepper (optional, for heat)
- 2 cans (15 oz each) chickpeas, rinsed and drained
- 1 can (14.5 oz) diced tomatoes (no salt added)
- 4 cups vegetable broth (low-sodium)
- 4 cups fresh spinach, roughly chopped
- Salt and pepper to taste
- 1/4 cup fresh cilantro or parsley, chopped (for garnish)
- 1 tablespoon lemon juice (optional, for added brightness)

Directions:

1. Sauté Aromatics: In a large pot, heat the olive oil over medium heat. Add the chopped onion and cook until softened, about 5 minutes. Add the minced garlic and cook for an additional 1-2 minutes until fragrant.

2. Add Spices: Stir in the ground cumin, ground coriander, smoked paprika, ground turmeric, and cayenne pepper (if using). Cook for 1-2 minutes to toast the spices and enhance their flavors.

3. Add Chickpeas and Tomatoes: Add the rinsed and drained chickpeas and the diced tomatoes to the pot. Stir well to combine.

4. Simmer Stew: Pour in the vegetable broth and bring the mixture to a boil. Reduce the heat to a simmer and cook for about 20 minutes, allowing the flavors to meld together.

5. Add Spinach: Stir in the roughly chopped fresh spinach. Cook for an additional 5 minutes, until the spinach is wilted and tender.

6. Season and Serve: Stir in the lemon juice (if using) and season with salt and pepper to taste. Ladle the stew into bowls and garnish with fresh cilantro or parsley. Serve hot.

Cooking Time:

Prep Time: 10 minutes
Cook Time: 30 minutes
Total Time: 40 minutes
Serving Size:

Serves 4
Nutritional Information (per serving):

Calories: 220
Protein: 10g
Carbohydrates: 30g
Dietary Fiber: 10g
Sugars: 6g
Fat: 8g

Saturated Fat: 1g
Vitamin A: 60% DV
Vitamin C: 30% DV
Calcium: 10% DV
Iron: 20% DV

9. Innovative Main Courses

9.1 Stuffed Bell Peppers with Quinoa and Vegetables

Ingredients:

- 4 large bell peppers (any color), tops cut off and seeds removed
- 1 cup quinoa, rinsed
- 2 cups vegetable broth (low-sodium)
- 2 tablespoons olive oil
- 1 large onion, chopped
- 3 cloves garlic, minced
- 1 zucchini, diced
- 1 cup cherry tomatoes, halved
- 1 can (15 oz) black beans, rinsed and drained
- 1 teaspoon ground cumin
- 1 teaspoon smoked paprika
- 1 teaspoon dried oregano
- Salt and pepper to taste
- 1/4 cup fresh parsley or cilantro, chopped
- 1/2 cup crumbled feta cheese (optional, for garnish)

Directions:

1. Preheat Oven: Preheat your oven to 375°F (190°C).

2. Cook Quinoa: In a medium saucepan, bring the vegetable broth to a boil. Add the rinsed quinoa, reduce the heat to low, cover, and simmer for about 15 minutes, or until the quinoa is cooked and the liquid is absorbed. Fluff with a fork and set aside.

3. Sauté Vegetables: In a large skillet, heat the olive oil over medium heat. Add the chopped onion and cook until softened, about 5 minutes. Add the minced garlic and cook for an additional 1-2 minutes until fragrant. Add the diced zucchini and cherry tomatoes, and cook for about 5-7 minutes until the vegetables are tender.

4. Combine Filling: Add the cooked quinoa, black beans, ground cumin, smoked paprika, and dried oregano to the skillet. Stir well to combine. Season with salt and pepper to taste. Stir in the chopped parsley or cilantro.

5. Stuff Bell Peppers: Place the hollowed bell peppers in a baking dish. Spoon the quinoa and vegetable mixture into each bell pepper, packing the filling tightly.

6. Bake: Cover the baking dish with aluminum foil and bake in the preheated oven for 25-30 minutes. Remove the foil and bake for an additional 10 minutes, until the bell peppers are tender and the tops are slightly browned.

7. Serve: Remove the stuffed peppers from the oven and let cool slightly. Garnish with crumbled feta cheese (if using) and additional fresh herbs. Serve warm.

Cooking Time:

Prep Time: 20 minutes
Cook Time: 45 minutes
Total Time: 1 hour 5 minutes
Serving Size:

Serves 4

Nutritional Information (per serving):

Calories: 350
Protein: 12g
Carbohydrates: 50g
Dietary Fiber: 12g
Sugars: 8g
Fat: 12g
Saturated Fat: 2g
Vitamin A: 100% DV
Vitamin C: 200% DV
Calcium: 15% DV
Iron: 20% DV

9.2 Eggplant Parmesan with Cashew Cheese

Ingredients:

- 2 large eggplants, sliced into 1/2-inch rounds
- 2 tablespoons olive oil
- Salt and pepper to taste
- 2 cups marinara sauce (low-histamine, homemade or store-bought)
- 1/2 cup fresh basil leaves, chopped

Cashew Cheese:

- 1 cup raw cashews, soaked in water for at least 2 hours
- 1/4 cup nutritional yeast
- 2 tablespoons lemon juice
- 1/2 teaspoon garlic powder
- 1/2 teaspoon onion powder
- Salt to taste
- 1/4 cup water (adjust for desired consistency)

Directions:

1. Prepare Cashew Cheese:

- Drain and rinse the soaked cashews. In a blender or food processor, combine the cashews, nutritional yeast, lemon juice, garlic powder, onion powder, salt, and water. Blend until smooth and creamy, adding more water if needed to achieve a cheese-like consistency. Set aside.

2. Preheat Oven:

- Preheat your oven to 400°F (200°C).

3. Prepare Eggplant:

- Arrange the eggplant slices on a baking sheet lined with parchment paper. Brush both sides of the eggplant slices with olive oil and season with salt and pepper.
- Bake in the preheated oven for 20-25 minutes, turning once halfway through, until the eggplant is tender and slightly golden.

4. Assemble Eggplant Parmesan:

- Reduce the oven temperature to 375°F (190°C).
- In a large baking dish, spread a thin layer of marinara sauce on the bottom. Place a layer of baked eggplant slices over the sauce. Spread a layer of cashew cheese over the eggplant, followed by a layer of marinara sauce. Repeat the layers until all ingredients are used, finishing with a layer of marinara sauce on top.

5. Bake:

- Cover the baking dish with aluminum foil and bake for 20 minutes. Remove the foil and bake for an additional 10 minutes, or until the top is bubbly and slightly golden.

6. Serve:

- Remove from the oven and let cool slightly. Garnish with chopped fresh basil leaves. Serve warm.

Cooking Time:

Prep Time: 20 minutes
Cook Time: 55 minutes
Total Time: 1 hour 15 minutes
Serving Size:

Serves 4

Nutritional Information (per serving):

Calories: 350

Protein: 10g

Carbohydrates: 40g

Dietary Fiber: 12g

Sugars: 10g

Fat: 18g

Saturated Fat: 3g

Vitamin A: 25% DV

Vitamin C: 35% DV

Calcium: 10% DV

Iron: 15% DV

9.3 Grilled Portobello Mushrooms with Balsamic Glaze

Ingredients:

- 4 large Portobello mushrooms, stems removed and wiped clean
- 3 tablespoons olive oil
- 3 tablespoons balsamic vinegar
- 2 cloves garlic, minced
- 1 teaspoon dried oregano
- Salt and pepper to taste
- Fresh parsley, chopped (for garnish)

Directions:

1. Prepare Marinade:

- In a small bowl, whisk together the olive oil, balsamic vinegar, minced garlic, dried oregano, salt, and pepper.

2. Marinate Mushrooms:

- Place the cleaned Portobello mushrooms in a shallow dish or a resealable plastic bag. Pour the marinade over the mushrooms, ensuring they are evenly coated. Let them marinate for at least 30 minutes, turning occasionally to ensure even marination.

3. Preheat Grill:

- Preheat your grill to medium-high heat (about 375°F to 400°F / 190°C to 200°C). If using a grill pan, preheat it over medium-high heat.

4. Grill Mushrooms:

- Remove the mushrooms from the marinade and place them on the preheated grill, gill side up. Reserve the marinade. Grill for about 5-7 minutes per side, or until the mushrooms are tender and have nice grill marks. Brush the mushrooms with the reserved marinade occasionally during grilling.

5. Prepare Balsamic Glaze (Optional):

- If you prefer a thicker balsamic glaze, pour the remaining marinade into a small saucepan and simmer over medium heat until it reduces and thickens, about 5-7 minutes.

6. Serve:

- Remove the mushrooms from the grill and let them rest for a few minutes. Slice the mushrooms and drizzle with the balsamic glaze, if prepared. Garnish with chopped fresh parsley. Serve warm.

Cooking Time:

Prep Time: 10 minutes (plus 30 minutes marinating time)
Cook Time: 15 minutes
Total Time: 55 minutes

Serving Size:

Serves 4

Nutritional Information (per serving):

Calories: 120
Protein: 3g
Carbohydrates: 10g
Dietary Fiber: 2g

Sugars: 6g

Fat: 8g

Saturated Fat: 1g

Vitamin A: 2% DV

Vitamin C: 10% DV

Calcium: 2% DV

Iron: 4% DV

9.4 Tofu Stir-Fry with Broccoli and Peppers

Ingredients:

- 1 block (14 oz) firm tofu, pressed and cubed
- 2 tablespoons olive oil, divided
- 2 cups broccoli florets
- 1 red bell pepper, sliced
- 1 yellow bell pepper, sliced
- 1 large carrot, julienned
- 3 cloves garlic, minced
- 1 tablespoon fresh ginger, minced
- 3 tablespoons low-sodium soy sauce or tamari (for gluten-free)
- 2 tablespoons rice vinegar
- 1 tablespoon maple syrup or honey
- 1 teaspoon cornstarch mixed with 2 tablespoons water
- 1/4 cup green onions, chopped
- 2 tablespoons sesame seeds (optional, for garnish)

Directions:

1. Press the tofu for at least 20 minutes to remove excess moisture. Cut the tofu into 1-inch cubes. In a large skillet or wok, heat 1 tablespoon of olive oil over medium-high heat. Add the cubed tofu and cook until golden brown on all sides, about 7-10 minutes. Remove the tofu from the skillet and set aside.

2. In the same skillet, add the remaining 1 tablespoon of olive oil. Add the minced garlic and ginger, and sauté for about 1 minute until fragrant. Add the broccoli florets, sliced red and yellow bell peppers, and julienned carrot. Stir-fry for about 5-7 minutes until the vegetables are tender-crisp.

3. In a small bowl, whisk together the soy sauce or tamari, rice vinegar, maple syrup or honey, and the cornstarch-water mixture. Return the cooked tofu to the skillet with the vegetables. Pour the sauce over the tofu and vegetables, stirring well to coat everything evenly. Cook for an additional 2-3 minutes until the sauce has thickened and everything is heated through.

4. Remove from heat and garnish with chopped green onions and sesame seeds (if using). Serve hot, over rice or noodles if desired.

Cooking Time:

Prep Time: 15 minutes (plus 20 minutes pressing tofu)
Cook Time: 20 minutes
Total Time: 35 minutes
Serving Size:

Serves 4
Nutritional Information (per serving):

Calories: 220
Protein: 10g
Carbohydrates: 20g
Dietary Fiber: 4g
Sugars: 8g
Fat: 12g
Saturated Fat: 2g
Vitamin A: 60% DV
Vitamin C: 150% DV
Calcium: 15% DV
Iron: 15% DV

9.5 Vegetable Paella with Saffron

Ingredients:

- 1 cup paella rice (Spanish short-grain rice)
- 2 tablespoons olive oil
- 1 onion, finely chopped
- 3 cloves garlic, minced
- 1 red bell pepper, diced
- 1 yellow bell pepper, diced
- 1 zucchini, diced
- 1 cup cherry tomatoes, halved
- 1 cup green beans, trimmed and cut into 1-inch pieces
- 1 teaspoon smoked paprika
- 1/2 teaspoon saffron threads
- 2 1/2 cups vegetable broth (low-sodium)
- Salt and pepper to taste
- 1/4 cup fresh parsley, chopped
- Lemon wedges, for serving

Directions:

1. In a small bowl, combine the saffron threads with 1 tablespoon of warm water and set aside.

2. In a large skillet or paella pan, heat the olive oil over medium heat. Add the chopped onion and cook until softened, about 5 minutes. Add the minced garlic and cook for an additional 1-2 minutes until fragrant.

3. Add the diced red and yellow bell peppers, diced zucchini, cherry tomatoes, and green beans to the skillet. Cook for about 5-7 minutes, stirring occasionally, until the vegetables start to soften.

4. Stir in the smoked paprika and paella rice, coating the rice with the oil and spices. Cook for 1-2 minutes to toast the rice slightly.

5. Pour in the vegetable broth and the saffron water mixture. Season with salt and pepper to taste. Bring to a boil, then reduce the heat to low. Simmer uncovered for 20-25 minutes, or until the rice is tender and most of the liquid has been absorbed. Avoid stirring the paella during this time to develop a crispy bottom layer (socarrat).

6. Remove the skillet from heat and let it rest, covered with a clean kitchen towel, for 5 minutes.

7. Garnish with chopped fresh parsley and serve with lemon wedges on the side for squeezing over the paella.

Cooking Time:

Prep Time: 15 minutes
Cook Time: 35 minutes
Total Time: 50 minutes
Serving Size:

Serves 4
Nutritional Information (per serving):

Calories: 300

Protein: 6g

Carbohydrates: 55g

Dietary Fiber: 6g

Sugars: 8g

Fat: 7g

Saturated Fat: 1g

Vitamin A: 60% DV

Vitamin C: 150% DV

Calcium: 6% DV

Iron: 15% DV

10. Comforting Pasta and Grain Dishes

10.1 Pesto Zucchini Noodles

Ingredients:

- 4 medium zucchinis
- 1/2 cup basil pesto (homemade or store-bought)
- 1 cup cherry tomatoes, halved
- 1/4 cup pine nuts, toasted
- Salt and pepper to taste
- Fresh basil leaves, thinly sliced (for garnish)
- Grated Parmesan cheese or nutritional yeast (optional, for serving)

Directions:

1. Using a spiralizer or a vegetable peeler, create zucchini noodles (zoodles) from the zucchinis. Set aside.

2. In a large skillet, heat the basil pesto over medium heat until warmed through, about 1-2 minutes.

3. Add the zucchini noodles to the skillet, tossing gently to coat them evenly with the pesto. Cook for 2-3 minutes, stirring occasionally, until the zucchini noodles are just tender.

4. Stir in the halved cherry tomatoes and toasted pine nuts. Cook for another 1-2 minutes until the tomatoes are heated through.

5. Season with salt and pepper to taste.

6. Remove from heat and garnish with thinly sliced fresh basil leaves.

7. Serve hot, optionally topped with grated Parmesan cheese or nutritional yeast.

Cooking Time:

Prep Time: 10 minutes
Cook Time: 5 minutes
Total Time: 15 minutes
Serving Size:

Serves 4
Nutritional Information (per serving):

Calories: 200
Protein: 5g
Carbohydrates: 10g
Dietary Fiber: 3g
Sugars: 5g
Fat: 15g
Saturated Fat: 2g
Vitamin A: 20% DV
Vitamin C: 40% DV
Calcium: 6% DV
Iron: 10% DV

10.2 Millet and Vegetable Stir-Fry

Ingredients:

- 1 cup millet, rinsed
- 2 cups water or vegetable broth
- 2 tablespoons olive oil
- 1 onion, chopped
- 2 cloves garlic, minced
- 1 red bell pepper, sliced
- 1 yellow bell pepper, sliced
- 1 cup broccoli florets
- 1 cup snow peas, trimmed
- 1 carrot, julienned
- 1/4 cup low-sodium soy sauce or tamari (for gluten-free)
- 2 tablespoons rice vinegar
- 1 tablespoon maple syrup or honey
- 1 tablespoon toasted sesame oil
- Salt and pepper to taste
- 1/4 cup chopped green onions (for garnish)
- Sesame seeds (optional, for garnish)

Directions:

1. In a medium saucepan, combine the rinsed millet and water or vegetable broth. Bring to a boil over high heat, then reduce the heat to low, cover, and simmer for 15-20 minutes, or until the millet is tender and all the liquid is absorbed. Remove from heat and let it sit covered for 5 minutes. Fluff with a fork and set aside.

2. In a large skillet or wok, heat the olive oil over medium-high heat. Add the chopped onion and minced garlic, and sauté for 2-3 minutes until the onion is translucent.

3. Add the sliced red and yellow bell peppers, broccoli florets, snow peas, and julienned carrot to the skillet. Stir-fry for about 5-7 minutes until the vegetables are tender-crisp.

4. In a small bowl, whisk together the soy sauce or tamari, rice vinegar, maple syrup or honey, and toasted sesame oil.

5. Add the cooked millet to the skillet with the stir-fried vegetables. Pour the sauce over the mixture and toss everything together gently to combine. Cook for an additional 2-3 minutes until heated through.

6. Season with salt and pepper to taste.

7. Remove from heat and garnish with chopped green onions and sesame seeds (if using).

8. Serve hot, optionally garnished with additional sesame seeds.

Cooking Time:

Prep Time: 10 minutes
Cook Time: 25 minutes
Total Time: 35 minutes
Serving Size:

Serves 4

Nutritional Information (per serving):

Calories: 350
Protein: 10g
Carbohydrates: 55g
Dietary Fiber: 8g
Sugars: 8g
Fat: 10g
Saturated Fat: 1g
Vitamin A: 120% DV
Vitamin C: 150% DV
Calcium: 8% DV
Iron: 20% DV

10.3 Quinoa Stuffed Tomatoes

Ingredients:

- 6 large tomatoes
- 1 cup quinoa, rinsed
- 2 cups vegetable broth or water
- 2 tablespoons olive oil
- 1 onion, finely chopped
- 2 cloves garlic, minced
- 1 red bell pepper, diced
- 1 yellow bell pepper, diced
- 1 zucchini, diced
- 1/2 cup corn kernels (fresh or frozen)
- 1/2 cup black beans, drained and rinsed
- 1 teaspoon ground cumin
- 1 teaspoon smoked paprika
- Salt and pepper to taste
- 1/4 cup fresh cilantro or parsley, chopped (for garnish)
- Lime wedges, for serving

Directions:

1. Preheat the oven to 375°F (190°C).

2. Cut the tops off the tomatoes and carefully scoop out the seeds and pulp using a spoon. Place the hollowed-out tomatoes in a baking dish, cut side up, and set aside.

3. In a medium saucepan, combine the quinoa and vegetable broth or water. Bring to a boil over high heat, then reduce the heat to low, cover, and simmer for 15

minutes, or until the quinoa is cooked and fluffy. Remove from heat and let it sit covered for 5 minutes. Fluff with a fork and set aside.

4. In a large skillet, heat the olive oil over medium heat. Add the chopped onion and sauté for 3-4 minutes until softened.

5. Add the minced garlic, diced red and yellow bell peppers, diced zucchini, corn kernels, and black beans to the skillet. Cook for about 5-7 minutes, stirring occasionally, until the vegetables are tender.

6. Stir in the ground cumin, smoked paprika, salt, and pepper to taste. Cook for an additional 1-2 minutes to toast the spices.

7. Remove the skillet from heat and stir in the cooked quinoa until well combined.

8. Spoon the quinoa mixture into the hollowed-out tomatoes, packing it tightly.

9. Bake in the preheated oven for 20-25 minutes, or until the tomatoes are tender and slightly wrinkled.

10. Remove from the oven and let cool slightly before serving.

11. Garnish with chopped fresh cilantro or parsley, and serve with lime wedges on the side for squeezing over the stuffed tomatoes.

Cooking Time:

Prep Time: 20 minutes
Cook Time: 45 minutes
Total Time: 1 hour 5 minutes

Serving Size:

Serves 6

Nutritional Information (per serving):

Calories: 250

Protein: 9g

Carbohydrates: 40g

Dietary Fiber: 8g

Sugars: 6g

Fat: 7g

Saturated Fat: 1g

Vitamin A: 40% DV

Vitamin C: 120% DV

Calcium: 6% DV

Iron: 20% DV

10.4 Spinach and Ricotta Stuffed Shells (Dairy-Free)

Ingredients:

- 20 jumbo pasta shells
- 1 tablespoon olive oil
- 1 onion, finely chopped
- 3 cloves garlic, minced
- 5 cups fresh spinach leaves, chopped
- 1 (14 oz) block firm tofu, drained and crumbled
- 1/2 cup nutritional yeast
- 1/4 cup fresh basil, chopped
- 1/4 cup fresh parsley, chopped
- 1 teaspoon dried oregano
- Salt and pepper to taste
- 1 (24 oz) jar marinara sauce (check for low-histamine ingredients)
- Fresh basil leaves, thinly sliced (for garnish)
- Nutritional yeast or vegan Parmesan cheese (optional, for serving)

Directions:

1. Preheat the oven to 375°F (190°C). Cook the jumbo pasta shells according to package instructions until al dente. Drain and set aside.

2. In a large skillet, heat the olive oil over medium heat. Add the chopped onion and sauté for 3-4 minutes until softened.

3. Add the minced garlic and chopped spinach to the skillet. Cook for about 3-4 minutes until the spinach wilts.

4. In a large mixing bowl, combine the crumbled tofu, nutritional yeast, chopped fresh basil, chopped fresh parsley, dried oregano, salt, and pepper. Add the sautéed spinach mixture and mix well to combine.

5. Spread a thin layer of marinara sauce on the bottom of a baking dish.

6. Stuff each cooked pasta shell with the tofu-spinach mixture and place them in the baking dish.

7. Pour the remaining marinara sauce evenly over the stuffed shells.

8. Cover the baking dish with aluminum foil and bake in the preheated oven for 25-30 minutes, until the sauce is bubbling and the shells are heated through.

9. Remove from the oven and let it cool slightly before serving.

10. Garnish with thinly sliced fresh basil leaves and sprinkle with nutritional yeast or vegan Parmesan cheese, if desired.

Cooking Time:

Prep Time: 30 minutes
Cook Time: 30 minutes
Total Time: 1 hour
Serving Size:

Serves 6
Nutritional Information (per serving):

Calories: 350

Protein: 20g

Carbohydrates: 45g

Dietary Fiber: 8g

Sugars: 8g

Fat: 10g

Saturated Fat: 2g

Vitamin A: 120% DV

Vitamin C: 50% DV

Calcium: 20% DV

Iron: 25% DV

10.5 Wild Rice and Mushroom Pilaf

Ingredients:

- 1 cup wild rice
- 2 cups vegetable broth or water
- 2 tablespoons olive oil
- 1 onion, finely chopped
- 3 cloves garlic, minced
- 8 oz cremini mushrooms, sliced
- 1/2 cup chopped celery
- 1/2 cup chopped carrots
- 1/4 cup chopped fresh parsley
- 1 teaspoon dried thyme
- Salt and pepper to taste
- 1/4 cup toasted pine nuts or sliced almonds (for garnish)
- Fresh parsley, chopped (for garnish)

Directions:

1. Rinse the wild rice under cold water. In a medium saucepan, combine the rinsed wild rice and vegetable broth or water. Bring to a boil over high heat, then reduce the heat to low, cover, and simmer for 40-45 minutes, or until the rice is tender and the liquid is absorbed. Remove from heat and let it sit covered for 5 minutes. Fluff with a fork and set aside.

2. In a large skillet, heat the olive oil over medium heat. Add the chopped onion and sauté for 3-4 minutes until softened.

3. Add the minced garlic and sliced cremini mushrooms to the skillet. Cook for about 5-7 minutes, stirring occasionally, until the mushrooms release their juices and start to brown.

4. Stir in the chopped celery and carrots. Cook for another 3-4 minutes until the vegetables are tender-crisp.

5. Add the cooked wild rice to the skillet with the sautéed vegetables. Stir in the chopped fresh parsley and dried thyme. Season with salt and pepper to taste. Cook for an additional 2-3 minutes to heat through and allow the flavors to blend.

6. Remove from heat and transfer the pilaf to a serving dish.

7. Garnish with toasted pine nuts or sliced almonds and chopped fresh parsley.

Cooking Time:

Prep Time: 15 minutes
Cook Time: 50 minutes
Total Time: 1 hour 5 minutes
Serving Size:

Serves 4
Nutritional Information (per serving):

Calories: 300
Protein: 8g
Carbohydrates: 45g
Dietary Fiber: 5g

Sugars: 3g

Fat: 10g

Saturated Fat: 1g

Vitamin A: 80% DV

Vitamin C: 10% DV

Calcium: 6% DV

Iron: 15% DV

Part V: Tempting Sides and Snacks

11. Flavorful Vegetable Sides

11.1 Roasted Cauliflower with Turmeric

Ingredients:

- 1 large head cauliflower, cut into florets
- 2 tablespoons olive oil
- 1 teaspoon ground turmeric
- 1 teaspoon ground cumin
- 1/2 teaspoon smoked paprika
- 1/2 teaspoon garlic powder
- Salt and pepper to taste
- 1 tablespoon lemon juice
- Fresh cilantro or parsley, chopped (for garnish)

Directions:

1. Preheat the oven to 425°F (220°C). Line a baking sheet with parchment paper or lightly grease it with olive oil.

2. In a large bowl, combine the cauliflower florets, olive oil, ground turmeric, ground cumin, smoked paprika, garlic powder, salt, and pepper. Toss well to coat the cauliflower evenly with the spices and oil.

3. Spread the cauliflower florets in a single layer on the prepared baking sheet.

4. Roast in the preheated oven for 25-30 minutes, or until the cauliflower is tender and golden brown, stirring halfway through the cooking time.

5. Remove from the oven and drizzle with lemon juice.

6. Garnish with chopped fresh cilantro or parsley.

7. Serve hot as a side dish or appetizer.

Cooking Time:

Prep Time: 10 minutes

Cook Time: 30 minutes

Total Time: 40 minutes

Serving Size:

Serves 4

Nutritional Information (per serving):

Calories: 110

Protein: 3g

Carbohydrates: 11g

Dietary Fiber: 4g

Sugars: 3g

Fat: 7g

Saturated Fat: 1g

Vitamin A: 4% DV

Vitamin C: 80% DV

Calcium: 4% DV

Iron: 8% DV

11.2 Steamed Asparagus with Lemon Zest

Ingredients:

- 1 lb fresh asparagus, trimmed
- 2 tablespoons olive oil
- Zest of 1 lemon
- 1 tablespoon lemon juice
- Salt and pepper to taste
- Fresh parsley, chopped (for garnish, optional)

Directions:

1. Fill a large pot with about an inch of water and bring to a boil. Place a steamer basket inside the pot.

2. Add the trimmed asparagus to the steamer basket, cover, and steam for 5-7 minutes, or until the asparagus is tender but still crisp.

3. While the asparagus is steaming, in a small bowl, combine the olive oil, lemon zest, lemon juice, salt, and pepper.

4. Once the asparagus is cooked, remove it from the steamer and transfer to a serving platter.

5. Drizzle the lemon and olive oil mixture over the steamed asparagus.

6. Toss gently to coat the asparagus evenly.

7. Garnish with chopped fresh parsley, if desired.

8. Serve hot as a side dish.

Cooking Time:

Prep Time: 5 minutes
Cook Time: 7 minutes
Total Time: 12 minutes
Serving Size:

Serves 4
Nutritional Information (per serving):

Calories: 80
Protein: 2g
Carbohydrates: 5g
Dietary Fiber: 2g
Sugars: 2g
Fat: 7g
Saturated Fat: 1g
Vitamin A: 15% DV
Vitamin C: 30% DV
Calcium: 4% DV
Iron: 10% DV

11.3 Sautéed Green Beans with Garlic

Ingredients:

- 1 lb fresh green beans, trimmed
- 2 tablespoons olive oil
- 3 cloves garlic, thinly sliced
- Salt and pepper to taste
- 1 tablespoon lemon juice (optional)
- 1/4 cup slivered almonds (optional, for garnish)
- Fresh parsley, chopped (for garnish, optional)

Directions:

1. Bring a large pot of salted water to a boil. Add the trimmed green beans and cook for 3-4 minutes, until bright green and tender-crisp. Drain and transfer immediately to a bowl of ice water to stop the cooking process. Drain again and set aside.

2. In a large skillet, heat the olive oil over medium heat. Add the thinly sliced garlic and sauté for 1-2 minutes, until fragrant and just beginning to turn golden.

3. Add the blanched green beans to the skillet and toss to coat them in the garlic-infused oil. Sauté for 4-5 minutes, stirring occasionally, until the green beans are heated through and slightly browned.

4. Season with salt and pepper to taste. If desired, drizzle with lemon juice for a bright, tangy flavor.

5. Transfer the sautéed green beans to a serving dish.

6. Garnish with slivered almonds and chopped fresh parsley, if using.

7. Serve hot as a side dish.

Cooking Time:

Prep Time: 10 minutes

Cook Time: 10 minutes

Total Time: 20 minutes

Serving Size:

Serves 4

Nutritional Information (per serving):

Calories: 120

Protein: 2g

Carbohydrates: 9g

Dietary Fiber: 4g

Sugars: 4g

Fat: 9g

Saturated Fat: 1g

Vitamin A: 15% DV

Vitamin C: 20% DV

Calcium: 4% DV

Iron: 6% DV

11.4 Grilled Zucchini with Herb Dressing

Ingredients:

- 4 medium zucchinis, sliced lengthwise into 1/4-inch thick strips
- 2 tablespoons olive oil
- Salt and pepper to taste
- 1 tablespoon balsamic vinegar
- 1 clove garlic, minced
- 2 tablespoons fresh parsley, chopped
- 2 tablespoons fresh basil, chopped
- 1 tablespoon fresh oregano, chopped
- 1 teaspoon lemon zest
- 1 tablespoon lemon juice

Directions:

1. Preheat the grill to medium-high heat.

2. Brush both sides of the zucchini strips with olive oil and season with salt and pepper.

3. Grill the zucchini strips for 2-3 minutes per side, or until tender and grill marks appear. Remove from the grill and set aside.

4. In a small bowl, whisk together the balsamic vinegar, minced garlic, chopped parsley, basil, oregano, lemon zest, and lemon juice.

5. Arrange the grilled zucchini strips on a serving platter.

6. Drizzle the herb dressing over the grilled zucchini.

7. Toss gently to coat the zucchini evenly with the dressing.

8. Serve warm or at room temperature as a side dish.

Cooking Time:

Prep Time: 10 minutes

Cook Time: 6 minutes

Total Time: 16 minutes

Serving Size:

Serves 4

Nutritional Information (per serving):

Calories: 90

Protein: 2g

Carbohydrates: 7g

Dietary Fiber: 2g

Sugars: 4g

Fat: 7g

Saturated Fat: 1g

Vitamin A: 10% DV

Vitamin C: 25% DV

Calcium: 4% DV

Iron: 6% DV

11.5 Baked Sweet Potato Fries

Ingredients:

- 2 large sweet potatoes, peeled and cut into thin strips
- 2 tablespoons olive oil
- 1 teaspoon paprika
- 1/2 teaspoon garlic powder
- 1/2 teaspoon salt
- 1/4 teaspoon black pepper
- 1/4 teaspoon cayenne pepper (optional, for a spicy kick)
- Fresh parsley, chopped (for garnish, optional)

Directions:

1. Preheat the oven to 425°F (220°C). Line a baking sheet with parchment paper or lightly grease it with olive oil.

2. In a large bowl, toss the sweet potato strips with olive oil, paprika, garlic powder, salt, black pepper, and cayenne pepper (if using) until evenly coated.

3. Spread the sweet potato strips in a single layer on the prepared baking sheet, ensuring they are not overcrowded. Use two baking sheets if necessary.

4. Bake in the preheated oven for 20-25 minutes, flipping halfway through, until the fries are tender and crispy on the edges.

5. Remove from the oven and transfer the fries to a serving platter.

6. Garnish with chopped fresh parsley, if desired.

7. Serve hot as a side dish or snack.

Cooking Time:

Prep Time: 10 minutes

Cook Time: 25 minutes

Total Time: 35 minutes

Serving Size:

Serves 4

Nutritional Information (per serving):

Calories: 160

Protein: 2g

Carbohydrates: 25g

Dietary Fiber: 4g

Sugars: 5g

Fat: 7g

Saturated Fat: 1g

Vitamin A: 370% DV

Vitamin C: 6% DV

Calcium: 4% DV

Iron: 6% DV

12. Healthy and Tasty Snacks

12.1 Baked Kale Chips

Ingredients:

- 1 bunch kale, washed and thoroughly dried
- 1 tablespoon olive oil
- 1/2 teaspoon salt
- 1/4 teaspoon garlic powder (optional)
- 1/4 teaspoon paprika (optional)

Directions:

1. Preheat the oven to 300°F (150°C). Line a baking sheet with parchment paper or lightly grease it with olive oil.

2. Remove the kale leaves from their thick stems and tear them into bite-sized pieces.

3. In a large bowl, toss the kale pieces with olive oil, salt, garlic powder, and paprika until evenly coated.

4. Spread the kale pieces in a single layer on the prepared baking sheet, ensuring they do not overlap.

5. Bake in the preheated oven for 20-25 minutes, or until the kale is crispy but not burnt. Check the kale chips frequently after 15 minutes to prevent burning.

6. Remove from the oven and let cool on the baking sheet for a few minutes.

7. Transfer the kale chips to a serving bowl.

8. Serve immediately as a healthy snack or appetizer.

Cooking Time:

Prep Time: 10 minutes
Cook Time: 25 minutes
Total Time: 35 minutes
Serving Size:

Serves 4
Nutritional Information (per serving):

Calories: 60
Protein: 2g
Carbohydrates: 5g
Dietary Fiber: 2g
Sugars: 0g
Fat: 4g
Saturated Fat: 1g
Vitamin A: 180% DV
Vitamin C: 80% DV
Calcium: 10% DV
Iron: 6% DV

12.2 Fresh Herb Guacamole with Veggie Sticks

Ingredients:

- 2 ripe avocados
- 1/4 cup finely chopped red onion
- 1 small tomato, diced
- 1/4 cup chopped fresh cilantro
- 1/4 cup chopped fresh parsley
- Juice of 1 lime
- Salt and pepper to taste
- Carrot sticks, cucumber sticks, and bell pepper strips (for serving)

Directions:

1. Cut the avocados in half, remove the pits, and scoop the flesh into a medium bowl.

2. Mash the avocados with a fork until smooth or leave slightly chunky, depending on your preference.

3. Add the finely chopped red onion, diced tomato, chopped cilantro, chopped parsley, and lime juice to the bowl with the mashed avocado.

4. Season with salt and pepper to taste. Mix until all ingredients are well combined.

5. Cover the guacamole with plastic wrap, pressing the wrap directly onto the surface to prevent browning, and refrigerate for at least 30 minutes to allow the flavors to meld.

6. Before serving, taste and adjust seasoning if needed.

7. Serve the fresh herb guacamole with carrot sticks, cucumber sticks, and bell pepper strips for dipping.

Cooking Time:

Prep Time: 15 minutes
Total Time: 15 minutes (plus chilling time)
Serving Size:

Serves 4
Nutritional Information (per serving, guacamole only):

Calories: 160
Protein: 2g
Carbohydrates: 9g
Dietary Fiber: 7g
Sugars: 1g
Fat: 14g
Saturated Fat: 2g
Vitamin A: 10% DV
Vitamin C: 20% DV
Calcium: 2% DV
Iron: 4% DV

12.3 Spiced Chickpeas

Ingredients:

- 2 cans (15 oz each) chickpeas, drained, rinsed, and patted dry
- 2 tablespoons olive oil
- 1 teaspoon ground cumin
- 1 teaspoon paprika
- 1/2 teaspoon ground coriander
- 1/2 teaspoon garlic powder
- 1/4 teaspoon cayenne pepper (adjust to taste)
- Salt to taste
- Fresh cilantro, chopped (for garnish, optional)
- Lemon wedges (for serving, optional)

Directions:

1. Preheat the oven to 400°F (200°C). Line a baking sheet with parchment paper or lightly grease it with olive oil.

2. In a large bowl, toss the chickpeas with olive oil, ground cumin, paprika, ground coriander, garlic powder, cayenne pepper, and salt until evenly coated.

3. Spread the seasoned chickpeas in a single layer on the prepared baking sheet.

4. Bake in the preheated oven for 25-30 minutes, stirring halfway through, until the chickpeas are crispy and golden brown.

5. Remove from the oven and let cool slightly on the baking sheet.

6. Transfer the spiced chickpeas to a serving bowl.

7. Garnish with chopped fresh cilantro, if desired, and serve with lemon wedges on the side for squeezing over the chickpeas.

Cooking Time:

Prep Time: 10 minutes
Cook Time: 25-30 minutes
Total Time: 35-40 minutes
Serving Size:

Serves 6
Nutritional Information (per serving):

Calories: 230
Protein: 9g
Carbohydrates: 32g
Dietary Fiber: 9g
Sugars: 6g
Fat: 8g
Saturated Fat: 1g
Sodium: 390mg
Potassium: 290mg
Vitamin A: 10% DV
Vitamin C: 4% DV
Calcium: 6% DV
Iron: 15% DV

12.4 Almond Butter Energy Balls

Ingredients:

- 1 cup rolled oats
- 1/2 cup almond butter
- 1/4 cup honey or maple syrup
- 1/4 cup ground flaxseed
- 1/4 cup mini chocolate chips (optional)
- 1 teaspoon vanilla extract
- 1/4 teaspoon salt
- 1/4 cup unsweetened shredded coconut (optional, for rolling)

Directions:

1. In a large mixing bowl, combine the rolled oats, almond butter, honey or maple syrup, ground flaxseed, mini chocolate chips (if using), vanilla extract, and salt. Mix well until all the ingredients are thoroughly combined.

2. Using your hands or a small cookie scoop, form the mixture into 1-inch balls. If the mixture is too sticky to handle, refrigerate it for 15-20 minutes before rolling.

3. Optional: Roll each energy ball in the shredded coconut to coat.

4. Place the energy balls on a baking sheet lined with parchment paper.

5. Refrigerate the energy balls for at least 30 minutes to firm up.

6. Once firm, transfer the energy balls to an airtight container and store in the refrigerator for up to 1 week.

Cooking Time:

Prep Time: 15 minutes

Chill Time: 30 minutes

Total Time: 45 minutes

Serving Size:

Makes approximately 20 energy balls

Nutritional Information (per energy ball):

Calories: 100

Protein: 3g

Carbohydrates: 10g

Dietary Fiber: 2g

Sugars: 6g

Fat: 6g

Saturated Fat: 1g

Vitamin A: 0% DV

Vitamin C: 0% DV

Calcium: 2% DV

Iron: 4% DV

12.5 Veggie Sushi Rolls

Ingredients:

- 2 cups sushi rice
- 2 1/2 cups water
- 1/4 cup rice vinegar
- 2 tablespoons sugar
- 1 teaspoon salt
- 4 sheets nori (seaweed)
- 1 small cucumber, julienned
- 1 small carrot, julienned
- 1 avocado, thinly sliced
- 1/2 red bell pepper, julienned
- 1/2 cup microgreens or sprouts
- Soy sauce (for serving)
- Pickled ginger (for serving)
- Wasabi (optional, for serving)

Directions:

1. Rinse the sushi rice under cold water until the water runs clear. Combine the rice and water in a medium saucepan and bring to a boil over medium-high heat.

2. Once boiling, reduce the heat to low, cover, and simmer for 18-20 minutes, or until the water is absorbed and the rice is tender.

3. Remove from heat and let the rice sit, covered, for 10 minutes. Transfer the rice to a large bowl.

4. In a small bowl, combine the rice vinegar, sugar, and salt. Microwave for 30 seconds, or until the sugar and salt are dissolved.

5. Pour the vinegar mixture over the rice and gently fold it in until the rice is evenly coated. Allow the rice to cool to room temperature.

6. Place a sheet of nori on a bamboo sushi mat, shiny side down.

7. Wet your hands with water to prevent sticking and spread a thin, even layer of sushi rice over the nori, leaving a 1-inch border at the top.

8. Arrange a few pieces of cucumber, carrot, avocado, bell pepper, and microgreens horizontally across the middle of the rice.

9. Using the bamboo mat, carefully roll the nori and rice over the filling, pressing gently but firmly to create a tight roll. Seal the edge with a little water if needed.

10. Repeat with the remaining nori sheets and fillings.

11. Using a sharp knife, cut each roll into 6-8 pieces.

12. Serve the veggie sushi rolls with soy sauce, pickled ginger, and wasabi (if using).

Cooking Time:

Prep Time: 30 minutes
Cook Time: 20 minutes
Total Time: 50 minutes

Serving Size:

Makes 4 rolls (24-32 pieces)
Nutritional Information (per piece):

Calories: 40
Protein: 1g
Carbohydrates: 8g
Dietary Fiber: 1g
Sugars: 1g
Fat: 1g
Saturated Fat: 0g
Vitamin A: 10% DV
Vitamin C: 8% DV
Calcium: 1% DV
Iron: 2% DV

Part VI: Decadent Desserts

13. Sweet Treats Without the Guilt

13.1 Coconut Milk Panna Cotta with Berries

Ingredients:

- 2 cups full-fat coconut milk
- 1/4 cup honey or maple syrup
- 1 teaspoon vanilla extract
- 2 1/2 teaspoons agar-agar powder (or 1 packet gelatin for a non-vegetarian option)
- Fresh berries (strawberries, blueberries, raspberries) for topping
- Fresh mint leaves for garnish (optional)

Directions:

1. In a small saucepan, combine the coconut milk, honey or maple syrup, and vanilla extract. Whisk until well blended.

2. Sprinkle the agar-agar powder over the mixture and whisk to combine. Let it sit for 5 minutes to allow the agar-agar to hydrate.

3. Place the saucepan over medium heat and bring the mixture to a gentle boil, stirring frequently. Continue to cook for 3-4 minutes, or until the agar-agar is completely dissolved.

4. Remove from heat and let the mixture cool slightly for 2-3 minutes.

5. Pour the mixture into 4 small ramekins or dessert cups.

6. Refrigerate the panna cotta for at least 2 hours, or until set.

7. Before serving, top each panna cotta with fresh berries and garnish with mint
    leaves if desired.

Serving Size:

Serves 4

Nutritional Information (per serving):

Calories: 230
Protein: 2g
Carbohydrates: 20g
Dietary Fiber: 1g
Sugars: 17g
Fat: 16g
Saturated Fat: 14g
Vitamin C: 15% DV
Calcium: 2% DV
Iron: 10% DV

13.2 Almond Flour Chocolate Chip Cookies

Ingredients:

- 2 cups almond flour
- 1/2 teaspoon baking soda
- 1/4 teaspoon salt
- 1/4 cup coconut oil, melted
- 1/4 cup honey or maple syrup
- 1 teaspoon vanilla extract
- 1/2 cup dark chocolate chips (dairy-free if needed)

Directions:

1. Preheat the oven to 350°F (175°C). Line a baking sheet with parchment paper.

2. In a medium bowl, whisk together the almond flour, baking soda, and salt.

3. In a separate bowl, combine the melted coconut oil, honey or maple syrup, and vanilla extract. Stir until well blended.

4. Pour the wet ingredients into the dry ingredients and mix until a dough forms.

5. Fold in the chocolate chips until evenly distributed throughout the dough.

6. Using a cookie scoop or tablespoon, drop rounded balls of dough onto the prepared baking sheet, spacing them about 2 inches apart.

7. Gently flatten each ball of dough with your fingers or the back of a spoon to form a cookie shape.

8. Bake in the preheated oven for 10-12 minutes, or until the edges are golden brown.

9. Remove from the oven and let the cookies cool on the baking sheet for 5 minutes before transferring them to a wire rack to cool completely.

Serving Size:

Makes approximately 12-14 cookies
Nutritional Information (per cookie):

Calories: 140
Protein: 3g
Carbohydrates: 12g
Dietary Fiber: 2g
Sugars: 8g
Fat: 10g
Saturated Fat: 4g
Vitamin E: 15% DV
Calcium: 4% DV
Iron: 6% DV

13.3 Avocado Chocolate Mousse

Ingredients:

- 2 ripe avocados
- 1/4 cup unsweetened cocoa powder
- 1/4 cup honey or maple syrup
- 1/4 cup almond milk (or other plant-based milk)
- 1 teaspoon vanilla extract
- Pinch of salt
- Fresh berries or mint leaves for garnish (optional)

Directions:

1. Cut the avocados in half, remove the pits, and scoop the flesh into a food processor or blender.

2. Add the cocoa powder, honey or maple syrup, almond milk, vanilla extract, and salt to the food processor.

3. Blend the ingredients until smooth and creamy, stopping to scrape down the sides as needed.

4. Taste the mousse and adjust the sweetness if necessary, adding more honey or maple syrup to taste.

5. Spoon the mousse into serving bowls or glasses.

6. Refrigerate for at least 30 minutes to allow the mousse to set and the flavors to meld.

7. Before serving, garnish with fresh berries or mint leaves if desired.

Serving Size:

Serves 4

Nutritional Information (per serving):

Calories: 210
Protein: 3g
Carbohydrates: 27g
Dietary Fiber: 7g
Sugars: 16g
Fat: 12g
Saturated Fat: 2g
Vitamin A: 4% DV
Vitamin C: 15% DV
Calcium: 4% DV
Iron: 10% DV

13.4 Lemon Coconut Bliss Balls

Ingredients:

- 1 cup almond flour
- 1 cup unsweetened shredded coconut
- 1/4 cup coconut oil, melted
- 1/4 cup honey or maple syrup
- Zest of 1 lemon
- Juice of 1 lemon
- 1 teaspoon vanilla extract
- Pinch of salt
- Extra shredded coconut for rolling (optional)

Directions:

1. In a large mixing bowl, combine the almond flour, shredded coconut, melted coconut oil, honey or maple syrup, lemon zest, lemon juice, vanilla extract, and salt. Mix until all ingredients are well combined and form a dough-like consistency.

2. Using your hands or a small cookie scoop, form the mixture into 1-inch balls.

3. If desired, roll each ball in additional shredded coconut to coat.

4. Place the bliss balls on a baking sheet lined with parchment paper.

5. Refrigerate the bliss balls for at least 30 minutes to firm up.

6. Once firm, transfer the bliss balls to an airtight container and store in the refrigerator for up to 1 week.

Serving Size:

Makes approximately 20 bliss balls
Nutritional Information (per bliss ball):

Calories: 100
Protein: 2g
Carbohydrates: 7g
Dietary Fiber: 2g
Sugars: 5g
Fat: 8g
Saturated Fat: 4g
Vitamin C: 4% DV
Calcium: 2% DV
Iron: 4% DV

13.5 Strawberry Chia Jam Bars

Ingredients:

For the Strawberry Chia Jam:

- 2 cups fresh strawberries, hulled and chopped
- 2 tablespoons honey or maple syrup
- 2 tablespoons chia seeds
- 1 teaspoon lemon juice

For the Crust and Topping:

- 1 1/2 cups almond flour
- 1/2 cup rolled oats
- 1/4 cup coconut oil, melted
- 1/4 cup honey or maple syrup
- 1 teaspoon vanilla extract
- Pinch of salt

Directions:

1. To Make the Strawberry Chia Jam:

- In a medium saucepan, combine the chopped strawberries and honey or maple syrup. Cook over medium heat, stirring occasionally, until the strawberries break down and become syrupy, about 10 minutes.

- Remove from heat and stir in the chia seeds and lemon juice. Let the mixture sit for 5-10 minutes to thicken, then set aside to cool.

2. To Make the Crust and Topping:

- Preheat the oven to 350°F (175°C). Line an 8x8-inch baking dish with parchment paper, leaving an overhang for easy removal.
-
- In a large bowl, mix together the almond flour, rolled oats, melted coconut oil, honey or maple syrup, vanilla extract, and salt until well combined.
-
- Press two-thirds of the mixture evenly into the bottom of the prepared baking dish to form the crust.
-
- Spread the cooled strawberry chia jam over the crust in an even layer.
-
- Sprinkle the remaining crust mixture over the top of the jam, pressing it gently to adhere.
-
- Bake in the preheated oven for 25-30 minutes, or until the top is golden brown.
-
- Remove from the oven and let the bars cool completely in the pan on a wire rack.
-
- Once cooled, use the parchment paper overhang to lift the bars out of the pan. Cut into squares and serve.

Serving Size:

Makes approximately 16 bars

Nutritional Information (per bar):

Calories: 130

Protein: 3g

Carbohydrates: 13g

Dietary Fiber: 3g

Sugars: 8g

Fat: 8g

Saturated Fat: 3g

Vitamin C: 10% DV

Calcium: 4% DV

Iron: 4% DV

14. Refreshing and Light Desserts

14.1 Mango Sorbet

Ingredients:

- 4 ripe mangoes, peeled and chopped
- 1/4 cup honey or maple syrup
- 1/4 cup water
- 1 tablespoon lime juice
- Pinch of salt

Directions:

1. Place the chopped mangoes in a blender or food processor and blend until smooth.

2. Add the honey or maple syrup, water, lime juice, and salt. Blend again until all the ingredients are well combined and smooth.

3. Pour the mixture into a shallow, freezer-safe container.

4. Freeze the mixture for about 2-3 hours, stirring every 30 minutes to break up any ice crystals and ensure a smooth texture.

5. Once fully frozen, let the sorbet sit at room temperature for 5-10 minutes before scooping to soften slightly.

6. Scoop the sorbet into bowls and serve immediately.

Serving Size:

Serves 4

Nutritional Information (per serving):

Calories: 120

Protein: 1g

Carbohydrates: 31g

Dietary Fiber: 3g

Sugars: 26g

Fat: 0.5g

Saturated Fat: 0g

Vitamin A: 30% DV

Vitamin C: 70% DV

Calcium: 2% DV

Iron: 2% DV

14.2 Chia Seed Pudding with Coconut and Mango

Ingredients:

- 1/4 cup chia seeds
- 1 cup coconut milk (from a can or carton)
- 1/4 cup water
- 2 tablespoons honey or maple syrup
- 1 teaspoon vanilla extract
- 1 ripe mango, peeled and diced
- Unsweetened shredded coconut for topping

Directions:

1. In a medium bowl, whisk together the chia seeds, coconut milk, water, honey or maple syrup, and vanilla extract until well combined.

2. Let the mixture sit for about 10 minutes, then whisk again to prevent the chia seeds from clumping together.

3. Cover the bowl and refrigerate for at least 2 hours, or overnight, until the chia seeds have absorbed the liquid and the mixture has thickened to a pudding-like consistency.

4. Before serving, give the chia seed pudding a good stir.

5. Divide the pudding into serving bowls or glasses.

6. Top each serving with the diced mango and a sprinkle of shredded coconut.

Serving Size:

Serves 4

Nutritional Information (per serving):

Calories: 220
Protein: 3g
Carbohydrates: 24g
Dietary Fiber: 6g
Sugars: 14g
Fat: 14g
Saturated Fat: 10g
Vitamin A: 15% DV
Vitamin C: 45% DV
Calcium: 10% DV
Iron: 15% DV

14.3 Fresh Fruit Salad with Mint

Ingredients:

- 1 cup strawberries, hulled and quartered
- 1 cup blueberries
- 1 cup pineapple, diced
- 1 cup mango, diced
- 1 cup kiwi, peeled and sliced
- 2 tablespoons fresh mint leaves, finely chopped
- 2 tablespoons honey or maple syrup (optional)
- 1 tablespoon lime juice

Directions:

1. In a large bowl, combine the strawberries, blueberries, pineapple, mango, and kiwi.

2. In a small bowl, whisk together the honey or maple syrup (if using) and lime juice.

3. Pour the lime juice mixture over the fruit and gently toss to coat.

4. Sprinkle the chopped mint leaves over the fruit salad and gently toss again to distribute the mint.

5. Chill the fruit salad in the refrigerator for at least 30 minutes to allow the flavors to meld.

6. Before serving, give the fruit salad a final toss and garnish with additional mint leaves if desired.

Serving Size:

Serves 4

Nutritional Information (per serving):

Calories: 100
Protein: 1g
Carbohydrates: 26g
Dietary Fiber: 4g
Sugars: 20g
Fat: 0.5g
Saturated Fat: 0g
Vitamin A: 10% DV
Vitamin C: 100% DV
Calcium: 4% DV
Iron: 4% DV

14.4 Apple Cinnamon Baked Chips

Ingredients:

- 3 large apples (Granny Smith, Honeycrisp, or Fuji are good choices)
- 1 teaspoon ground cinnamon
- 1 tablespoon coconut sugar or granulated sugar (optional)

Directions:

1. Preheat your oven to 225°F (110°C). Line two baking sheets with parchment paper.

2. Wash and core the apples. Using a mandoline slicer or a sharp knife, slice the apples as thinly as possible (about 1/8 inch thick).

3. Lay the apple slices in a single layer on the prepared baking sheets. Make sure the slices do not overlap.

4. In a small bowl, mix the ground cinnamon and coconut sugar (if using).

5. Sprinkle the cinnamon mixture evenly over the apple slices.

6. Bake the apple slices in the preheated oven for 1 hour, then flip the slices and bake for an additional 1-1.5 hours, or until the apples are dry and crispy.

7. Turn off the oven and let the apple chips cool in the oven for an additional hour to ensure they become fully crispy.

8. Once cooled, remove the apple chips from the oven and store them in an airtight container.

Serving Size:

Serves 4
Nutritional Information (per serving):

Calories: 60
Protein: 0.5g
Carbohydrates: 16g
Dietary Fiber: 3g
Sugars: 12g
Fat: 0g
Saturated Fat: 0g
Vitamin A: 2% DV
Vitamin C: 6% DV
Calcium: 2% DV
Iron: 2% DV

14.5 Raspberry Coconut Popsicles

Ingredients:

- 2 cups fresh or frozen raspberries
- 1 cup coconut milk (from a can or carton)
- 1/4 cup honey or maple syrup
- 1 teaspoon vanilla extract
- 1/4 cup unsweetened shredded coconut

Directions:

1. In a blender, combine the raspberries, coconut milk, honey or maple syrup, and vanilla extract. Blend until smooth.

2. Pour the raspberry mixture through a fine mesh strainer into a bowl to remove the seeds, pressing down with a spoon to extract as much liquid as possible.

3. Stir in the shredded coconut.

4. Pour the mixture into popsicle molds, leaving a little space at the top for expansion.

5. Insert popsicle sticks into each mold.

6. Freeze the popsicles for at least 4 hours, or until completely solid.

7. To release the popsicles, run warm water over the outside of the molds for a few seconds, then gently pull the popsicles out.

Serving Size:

Makes approximately 6 popsicles
Nutritional Information (per popsicle):

Calories: 90
Protein: 1g
Carbohydrates: 14g
Dietary Fiber: 3g
Sugars: 10g
Fat: 4g
Saturated Fat: 3g
Vitamin C: 15% DV
Calcium: 2% DV
Iron: 4% DV

Part VII: Sauces, Dips, and Condiments

15. Versatile and Flavorful Sauces

15.1 Low-Histamine Tomato Sauce

Ingredients:

- 2 cups fresh tomatoes, peeled and chopped (use low-histamine varieties like Roma or vine-ripened)
- 2 tablespoons extra virgin olive oil
- 1/2 cup water
- 1 small carrot, finely grated
- 1 stalk celery, finely chopped
- 1/2 small onion, finely chopped
- 2 cloves garlic, minced
- 1/4 teaspoon sea salt (or to taste)
- 1/4 teaspoon freshly ground black pepper (optional)
- 1/4 cup fresh basil leaves, chopped
- 1 teaspoon fresh oregano, chopped (optional)

Directions:

1. Prepare the Vegetables: Peel and chop the tomatoes. Finely grate the carrot, chop the celery and onion, and mince the garlic.

2. Sauté the Vegetables: In a large saucepan, heat the olive oil over medium heat. Add the onion, celery, and carrot, and sauté for about 5 minutes, or until the vegetables are softened.

3. Add Garlic: Add the minced garlic and sauté for another 1-2 minutes until fragrant, being careful not to burn the garlic.

4. Cook the Tomatoes: Add the chopped tomatoes to the saucepan and stir to combine with the vegetables. Add the water, salt, and pepper (if using). Bring the mixture to a simmer.

5. Simmer: Reduce the heat to low and let the sauce simmer for about 30-40 minutes, stirring occasionally, until the tomatoes are broken down and the sauce has thickened.

6. Blend the Sauce: If you prefer a smooth sauce, use an immersion blender to blend the sauce until smooth. Alternatively, you can transfer the sauce to a blender and blend until smooth, then return it to the saucepan.

7. Add Herbs: Stir in the chopped basil and oregano (if using). Simmer for another 5 minutes to allow the flavors to meld.

8. Adjust Seasoning: Taste the sauce and adjust the seasoning with additional salt and pepper if needed.

9. Serve or Store: Serve the sauce immediately over your favorite low-histamine pasta or vegetables, or let it cool and store it in airtight containers in the refrigerator for up to one week or freeze for longer storage.

Serving Size:

Makes approximately 4 servings

Nutritional Information (per serving):

Calories: 80

Protein: 1g

Carbohydrates: 8g

Dietary Fiber: 2g

Sugars: 5g

Fat: 5g

Saturated Fat: 1g

Vitamin A: 15% DV

Vitamin C: 30% DV

Calcium: 4% DV

Iron: 4% DV

15.2 Basil Pesto without Nuts

Ingredients:

- 2 cups fresh basil leaves, packed
- 1/2 cup extra virgin olive oil
- 1/4 cup grated Parmesan cheese (optional for dairy-free: use nutritional yeast)
- 2 cloves garlic, minced
- 1/4 teaspoon sea salt (or to taste)
- 1/4 teaspoon freshly ground black pepper (optional)
- 1 tablespoon lemon juice

Directions:

1. Prepare the Ingredients: Wash and dry the basil leaves thoroughly. Mince the garlic cloves.

2. Blend the Ingredients: In a food processor or blender, combine the basil leaves, garlic, lemon juice, salt, and pepper (if using).

3. Add the Olive Oil: While the food processor or blender is running, slowly drizzle in the olive oil until the mixture is smooth and well combined.

4. Add Cheese or Nutritional Yeast: Add the grated Parmesan cheese or nutritional yeast to the mixture and blend again until fully incorporated. Taste and adjust the seasoning as needed.

5. Store or Serve: Transfer the pesto to an airtight container. It can be used immediately or stored in the refrigerator for up to one week. For longer storage, you can freeze the pesto in ice cube trays and transfer the frozen cubes to a freezer-safe bag.

Serving Size:

Makes approximately 1 cup (serves 4)
Nutritional Information (per serving):

Calories: 200

Protein: 2g

Carbohydrates: 2g

Dietary Fiber: 1g

Sugars: 0g

Fat: 21g

Saturated Fat: 3g

Vitamin A: 15% DV

Vitamin C: 10% DV

Calcium: 10% DV

Iron: 8% DV

15.3 Lemon Herb Vinaigrette

Ingredients:

- 1/4 cup fresh lemon juice (about 2 lemons)
- 1/2 cup extra virgin olive oil
- 1 tablespoon Dijon mustard
- 1 tablespoon honey or maple syrup
- 1 clove garlic, minced
- 1 teaspoon fresh thyme leaves, chopped (or 1/2 teaspoon dried thyme)
- 1 teaspoon fresh oregano leaves, chopped (or 1/2 teaspoon dried oregano)
- 1/2 teaspoon sea salt (or to taste)
- 1/4 teaspoon freshly ground black pepper (optional)

Directions:

1. Prepare the Ingredients: Juice the lemons to yield about 1/4 cup of lemon juice. Mince the garlic. Chop the fresh thyme and oregano leaves if using fresh herbs.

2. Combine the Ingredients: In a small bowl or a jar with a tight-fitting lid, combine the lemon juice, Dijon mustard, honey or maple syrup, minced garlic, chopped thyme, chopped oregano, salt, and pepper.

3. Mix the Vinaigrette: Whisk the ingredients together until well combined. If using a jar, you can shake it vigorously to combine the ingredients.

4. Add the Olive Oil: Slowly drizzle in the olive oil while continuing to whisk, or if using a jar, add the olive oil and shake until the vinaigrette is well emulsified and smooth.

5. Adjust Seasoning: Taste the vinaigrette and adjust the seasoning with additional salt, pepper, or lemon juice if needed.

6. Store or Serve: Use immediately on salads or as a marinade. Store any leftovers in the refrigerator for up to one week. Shake or whisk well before each use as the ingredients may separate.

Serving Size:

Makes approximately 3/4 cup (serves 6)
Nutritional Information (per serving, approximately 2 tablespoons):

Calories: 140
Protein: 0g
Carbohydrates: 2g
Dietary Fiber: 0g
Sugars: 1g
Fat: 14g
Saturated Fat: 2g
Vitamin C: 6% DV
Calcium: 1% DV
Iron: 1% DV

15.4 Creamy Tahini Dressing

Ingredients:

- 1/4 cup tahini
- 1/4 cup water (more if needed)
- 2 tablespoons lemon juice (about 1 lemon)
- 1 tablespoon extra virgin olive oil
- 1 tablespoon maple syrup or honey
- 1 clove garlic, minced
- 1/2 teaspoon sea salt (or to taste)
- 1/4 teaspoon ground cumin (optional)
- 1/4 teaspoon freshly ground black pepper (optional)

Directions:

1. Prepare the Ingredients: Juice the lemon to yield about 2 tablespoons of lemon juice. Mince the garlic.

2. Combine Tahini and Lemon Juice: In a medium bowl, whisk together the tahini and lemon juice. The mixture will thicken initially.

3. Add Water: Gradually add water, a tablespoon at a time, whisking continuously until the dressing reaches your desired consistency. You may need to add a bit more water for a thinner dressing.

4. Add Remaining Ingredients: Whisk in the olive oil, maple syrup or honey, minced garlic, sea salt, ground cumin (if using), and black pepper (if using) until the dressing is smooth and well combined.

5. Adjust Seasoning: Taste the dressing and adjust the seasoning with additional salt, lemon juice, or maple syrup/honey as needed.

6. Store or Serve: Use immediately on salads, grain bowls, or as a dip for vegetables. Store any leftovers in an airtight container in the refrigerator for up to one week. Stir well before each use as the ingredients may separate.

Serving Size:

Makes approximately 1/2 cup (serves 4)

Nutritional Information (per serving, approximately 2 tablespoons):

Calories: 120
Protein: 3g
Carbohydrates: 6g
Dietary Fiber: 1g
Sugars: 4g
Fat: 10g
Saturated Fat: 1.5g
Vitamin C: 4% DV
Calcium: 4% DV
Iron: 6% DV

15.5 Roasted Red Pepper Sauce

Ingredients:

- 2 large red bell peppers
- 2 tablespoons extra virgin olive oil
- 1 clove garlic, minced
- 1/4 cup vegetable broth or water
- 1 tablespoon lemon juice
- 1 teaspoon apple cider vinegar
- 1/2 teaspoon sea salt (or to taste)
- 1/4 teaspoon freshly ground black pepper (optional)
- 1/4 teaspoon smoked paprika (optional for added depth of flavor)

Directions:

1. Roast the Peppers: Preheat your oven to 450°F (230°C). Place the whole red bell peppers on a baking sheet lined with parchment paper. Roast for 20-25 minutes, turning occasionally, until the skins are charred and blistered.

2. Steam and Peel the Peppers: Remove the peppers from the oven and place them in a bowl. Cover the bowl with plastic wrap or a plate to let the peppers steam for about 10 minutes. This will make the skins easier to peel off. Once steamed, peel off the skins, remove the seeds and stems, and set the roasted peppers aside.

3. Prepare the Ingredients: Mince the garlic.

4. Blend the Ingredients: In a blender or food processor, combine the roasted red peppers, minced garlic, vegetable broth or water, lemon juice, apple cider vinegar, sea salt, black pepper (if using), and smoked paprika (if using). Blend until smooth and creamy.

5. Adjust Consistency: If the sauce is too thick, add a bit more vegetable broth or water, one tablespoon at a time, until you reach your desired consistency.

6. Store or Serve: Use immediately as a sauce for pasta, grain bowls, or roasted vegetables. Store any leftovers in an airtight container in the refrigerator for up to one week. Stir well before each use.

Serving Size:

Makes approximately 1 cup (serves 4)
Nutritional Information (per serving, approximately 1/4 cup):

Calories: 50
Protein: 1g
Carbohydrates: 4g
Dietary Fiber: 1g
Sugars: 3g
Fat: 4g
Saturated Fat: 0.5g
Vitamin C: 80% DV
Vitamin A: 20% DV
Calcium: 1% DV
Iron: 2% DV

16. Dips and Spreads for Every Occasion

16.1 Creamy Avocado Dip

Ingredients:

- 2 ripe avocados
- 1/4 cup Greek yogurt or dairy-free yogurt (optional for creaminess)
- 1 tablespoon fresh lime juice (about 1 lime)
- 1 small clove garlic, minced
- 1 tablespoon fresh cilantro, chopped (optional)
- 1/4 teaspoon sea salt (or to taste)
- 1/4 teaspoon freshly ground black pepper (optional)
- 1/4 teaspoon ground cumin (optional for added flavor)

Directions:

1. Prepare the Ingredients: Cut the avocados in half, remove the pits, and scoop the flesh into a medium bowl. Mince the garlic and chop the cilantro if using.

2. Mash the Avocados: Using a fork or potato masher, mash the avocados until smooth and creamy.

3. Combine Ingredients: Add the Greek yogurt (if using), lime juice, minced garlic, chopped cilantro (if using), sea salt, black pepper (if using), and ground cumin (if using) to the mashed avocados.

4. Mix Well: Stir the ingredients together until well combined and smooth. Taste and adjust the seasoning with more salt, lime juice, or cumin as needed.

5. Store or Serve: Serve the creamy avocado dip immediately with vegetable sticks, tortilla chips, or use as a spread on sandwiches and wraps. Store any leftovers in an airtight container in the refrigerator for up to two days. To prevent browning, press plastic wrap directly onto the surface of the dip before sealing the container.

Serving Size:

Makes approximately 1 1/2 cups (serves 6)
Nutritional Information (per serving, approximately 1/4 cup):

Calories: 80
Protein: 1g
Carbohydrates: 5g
Dietary Fiber: 4g
Sugars: 1g
Fat: 7g
Saturated Fat: 1g
Vitamin C: 15% DV
Vitamin K: 10% DV
Folate: 10% DV
Potassium: 6% DV

16.2 Roasted Red Pepper Hummus

Ingredients:

- 1 can (15 ounces) chickpeas, drained and rinsed
- 1 large red bell pepper
- 1/4 cup tahini
- 2 tablespoons lemon juice (about 1 lemon)
- 2 tablespoons extra virgin olive oil
- 1 clove garlic, minced
- 1/2 teaspoon sea salt (or to taste)
- 1/4 teaspoon ground cumin (optional)
- 2-4 tablespoons water (to achieve desired consistency)
- Paprika or chopped fresh parsley for garnish (optional)

Directions:

1. Roast the Red Pepper: Preheat your oven to 450°F (230°C). Place the whole red bell pepper on a baking sheet lined with parchment paper. Roast for 20-25 minutes, turning occasionally, until the skin is charred and blistered. Remove from the oven and place the pepper in a bowl. Cover with plastic wrap or a plate to steam for about 10 minutes. Peel off the skin, remove the seeds and stem, and set the roasted pepper aside.

2. Prepare the Ingredients: Drain and rinse the chickpeas. Mince the garlic.

3. Blend the Ingredients: In a food processor or blender, combine the chickpeas, roasted red pepper, tahini, lemon juice, olive oil, minced garlic, sea salt, and cumin (if using). Blend until smooth.

4. Adjust Consistency: If the hummus is too thick, add water, one tablespoon at a time, blending until you reach the desired consistency.

5. Taste and Adjust: Taste the hummus and adjust the seasoning with additional salt, lemon juice, or cumin as needed.

6. Garnish and Serve: Transfer the hummus to a serving bowl. Drizzle with a little olive oil and sprinkle with paprika or chopped fresh parsley if desired. Serve with vegetable sticks, pita chips, or use as a spread in sandwiches and wraps.

7. Store Leftovers: Store any leftovers in an airtight container in the refrigerator for up to one week. Stir well before each use.

Serving Size:

Makes approximately 2 cups (serves 8)
Nutritional Information (per serving, approximately 1/4 cup):

Calories: 90
Protein: 3g
Carbohydrates: 8g
Dietary Fiber: 2g
Sugars: 1g
Fat: 5g
Saturated Fat: 1g
Vitamin C: 20% DV
Vitamin A: 10% DV
Calcium: 3% DV
Iron: 6% DV

16.3 White Bean and Rosemary Spread

Ingredients:

- 1 can (15 ounces) cannellini beans or other white beans, drained and rinsed
- 2 tablespoons extra virgin olive oil
- 2 tablespoons lemon juice (about 1 lemon)
- 1 clove garlic, minced
- 1 tablespoon fresh rosemary, finely chopped (or 1 teaspoon dried rosemary)
- 1/2 teaspoon sea salt (or to taste)
- 1/4 teaspoon freshly ground black pepper (optional)
- 2-4 tablespoons water (to achieve desired consistency)

Directions:

1. Prepare the Ingredients: Drain and rinse the white beans. Mince the garlic and finely chop the fresh rosemary if using.

2. Blend the Ingredients: In a food processor or blender, combine the white beans, olive oil, lemon juice, minced garlic, chopped rosemary, sea salt, and black pepper (if using). Blend until smooth and creamy.

3. Adjust Consistency: If the spread is too thick, add water, one tablespoon at a time, blending until you reach the desired consistency.

4. Taste and Adjust: Taste the spread and adjust the seasoning with additional salt, lemon juice, or rosemary as needed.

5. Store or Serve: Transfer the spread to a serving bowl. Serve with vegetable sticks, crackers, or use as a spread on sandwiches and wraps. Store any leftovers in an airtight container in the refrigerator for up to one week. Stir well before each use.

Serving Size:

Makes approximately 1 1/2 cups (serves 6)

Nutritional Information (per serving, approximately 1/4 cup):

Calories: 90

Protein: 3g

Carbohydrates: 10g

Dietary Fiber: 3g

Sugars: 0g

Fat: 4g

Saturated Fat: 0.5g

Vitamin C: 4% DV

Calcium: 4% DV

Iron: 8% DV

16.4 Carrot Ginger Dip

Ingredients:

- 2 large carrots, peeled and chopped
- 1/4 cup tahini
- 2 tablespoons fresh lemon juice (about 1 lemon)
- 1 tablespoon fresh ginger, grated
- 1 clove garlic, minced
- 2 tablespoons extra virgin olive oil
- 1/2 teaspoon ground cumin
- 1/2 teaspoon sea salt (or to taste)
- 2-4 tablespoons water (to achieve desired consistency)
- Fresh cilantro or parsley for garnish (optional)

Directions:

1. Prepare the Ingredients: Peel and chop the carrots. Grate the fresh ginger and mince the garlic.

2. Steam the Carrots: Place the chopped carrots in a steamer basket over boiling water. Steam for 8-10 minutes or until the carrots are tender when pierced with a fork. Remove from heat and let cool slightly.

3. Blend the Ingredients: In a food processor or blender, combine the steamed carrots, tahini, lemon juice, grated ginger, minced garlic, olive oil, ground cumin, and sea salt. Blend until smooth and creamy.

4. Adjust Consistency: If the dip is too thick, add water, one tablespoon at a time, blending until you reach the desired consistency.

5. Taste and Adjust: Taste the dip and adjust the seasoning with additional salt or lemon juice as needed.

6. Serve: Transfer the carrot ginger dip to a serving bowl. Garnish with fresh cilantro or parsley if desired. Serve with vegetable sticks, pita chips, or use as a spread on sandwiches and wraps.

7. Store Leftovers: Store any leftovers in an airtight container in the refrigerator for up to one week. Stir well before each use.

Serving Size:

Makes approximately 1 1/2 cups (serves 6)
Nutritional Information (per serving, approximately 1/4 cup):

Calories: 120
Protein: 3g
Carbohydrates: 8g
Dietary Fiber: 3g
Sugars: 2g
Fat: 9g
Saturated Fat: 1g
Vitamin A: 190% DV
Vitamin C: 10% DV
Calcium: 6% DV
Iron: 6% DV

16.5 Cashew Ricotta Cheese

Ingredients:

- 1 cup raw cashews, soaked in water for 4-6 hours or overnight
- 2 tablespoons nutritional yeast
- 2 tablespoons fresh lemon juice (about 1 lemon)
- 1 clove garlic, minced
- 1/2 teaspoon sea salt (or to taste)
- 1/4 cup water (more if needed for blending)
- Fresh basil or parsley, chopped (optional for garnish)

Directions:

1. Soak the Cashews: Place the raw cashews in a bowl and cover with water. Let them soak for 4-6 hours or overnight. Drain and rinse thoroughly before using.

2. Blend the Ingredients: In a food processor or high-speed blender, combine the soaked cashews, nutritional yeast, fresh lemon juice, minced garlic, sea salt, and water. Blend until smooth and creamy, scraping down the sides of the blender as needed. Add more water, a tablespoon at a time, if needed to achieve a creamy consistency.

3. Adjust Consistency and Seasoning: Taste the cashew ricotta and adjust the seasoning with more salt or lemon juice as desired. If the mixture is too thick, add a little more water and blend again until smooth.

4. Serve or Store: Transfer the cashew ricotta cheese to a serving bowl. Garnish with chopped fresh basil or parsley if desired. Use immediately as a spread on toast, in pasta dishes, or as a filling for wraps and sandwiches. Store any leftovers in an airtight container in the refrigerator for up to one week.

Serving Size:

Makes approximately 1 cup (serves 4)
Nutritional Information (per serving, approximately 1/4 cup):

Calories: 180
Protein: 6g
Carbohydrates: 10g
Dietary Fiber: 2g
Sugars: 2g
Fat: 14g
Saturated Fat: 2.5g
Vitamin C: 4% DV
Calcium: 2% DV
Iron: 10% DV

Part VIII: Beverages to Refresh and Rehydrate

17. Infused Waters and Herbal Teas

17.1 Cucumber Mint Infused Water

Ingredients:

- 1 medium cucumber
- 1 small bunch of fresh mint leaves (about 10-12 leaves)
- 8 cups (2 liters) cold water
- Ice cubes (optional)

Directions:

1. Prepare the Ingredients: Wash the cucumber and mint leaves thoroughly. Thinly slice the cucumber.

2. Combine Ingredients: In a large pitcher, add the cucumber slices and fresh mint leaves.

3. Add Water: Pour the cold water over the cucumber and mint.

4. Infuse: Allow the mixture to sit in the refrigerator for at least 2 hours to let the flavors meld. For a stronger flavor, let it infuse overnight.

5. Serve: Serve chilled over ice cubes if desired. Garnish with additional cucumber slices or mint leaves for presentation.

6. Store: Keep any leftovers in the refrigerator and consume within 2 days for the best flavor.

Serving Size:

Makes approximately 8 servings (1 cup per serving)
Nutritional Information (per serving):

Calories: 0
Protein: 0g
Carbohydrates: 0g
Dietary Fiber: 0g
Sugars: 0g
Fat: 0g
Saturated Fat: 0g
Sodium: 0mg
Vitamin C: 2% DV (from mint)
Calcium: 0% DV
Iron: 0% DV

17.2 Ginger and Turmeric Herbal Tea

Ingredients:

- 1 inch fresh ginger root, peeled and thinly sliced
- 1 inch fresh turmeric root, peeled and thinly sliced (or 1 teaspoon ground turmeric)
- 4 cups water
- 1 tablespoon fresh lemon juice (optional)
- 1-2 teaspoons honey or maple syrup (optional, for sweetness)

Directions:

1. Prepare the Ingredients: Peel and thinly slice the fresh ginger and turmeric roots.

2. Boil the Water: In a medium saucepan, bring 4 cups of water to a boil.

3. Add Ginger and Turmeric: Once the water is boiling, add the sliced ginger and turmeric. Reduce the heat and let it simmer for about 10-15 minutes.

4. Strain the Tea: After simmering, remove the saucepan from the heat. Strain the tea into a teapot or directly into cups to remove the ginger and turmeric pieces.

5. Add Lemon and Sweetener (Optional): Stir in the fresh lemon juice and honey or maple syrup if desired.

6. Serve: Pour the tea into cups and enjoy it hot. You can also let it cool and serve it over ice for a refreshing iced tea.

7. Store: Store any leftover tea in an airtight container in the refrigerator for up to 2 days. Reheat or serve chilled.

Serving Size:

Makes approximately 4 servings (1 cup per serving)
Nutritional Information (per serving, without optional ingredients):

Calories: 5
Protein: 0g
Carbohydrates: 1g
Dietary Fiber: 0g
Sugars: 0g
Fat: 0g
Saturated Fat: 0g
Vitamin C: 2% DV (if lemon juice is added)
Calcium: 1% DV
Iron: 1% DV

17.3 Lemon Basil Infused Water

Ingredients:

- 1 large lemon
- 1 small bunch of fresh basil leaves (about 10-12 leaves)
- 8 cups (2 liters) cold water
- Ice cubes (optional)

Directions:

1. Prepare the Ingredients: Wash the lemon and basil leaves thoroughly. Thinly slice the lemon.

2. Combine Ingredients: In a large pitcher, add the lemon slices and fresh basil leaves.

3. Add Water: Pour the cold water over the lemon and basil.

4. Infuse: Allow the mixture to sit in the refrigerator for at least 2 hours to let the flavors meld. For a stronger flavor, let it infuse overnight.

5. Serve: Serve chilled over ice cubes if desired. Garnish with additional lemon slices or basil leaves for presentation.

6. Store: Keep any leftovers in the refrigerator and consume within 2 days for the best flavor.

Serving Size:

Makes approximately 8 servings (1 cup per serving)

Nutritional Information (per serving):

Calories: 0
Protein: 0g
Carbohydrates: 0g
Dietary Fiber: 0g
Sugars: 0g
Fat: 0g
Saturated Fat: 0g
Sodium: 0mg
Vitamin C: 4% DV (from lemon)
Calcium: 0% DV
Iron: 0% DV

17.4 Hibiscus and Rose Hip Tea

Ingredients:

- 1 large lemon
- 1 small bunch of fresh basil leaves (about 10-12 leaves)
- 8 cups (2 liters) cold water
- Ice cubes (optional)

Directions:

1. Prepare the Ingredients: Wash the lemon and basil leaves thoroughly. Thinly slice the lemon.

2. Combine Ingredients: In a large pitcher, add the lemon slices and fresh basil leaves.

3. Add Water: Pour the cold water over the lemon and basil.

4. Infuse: Allow the mixture to sit in the refrigerator for at least 2 hours to let the flavors meld. For a stronger flavor, let it infuse overnight.

5. Serve: Serve chilled over ice cubes if desired. Garnish with additional lemon slices or basil leaves for presentation.

6. Store: Keep any leftovers in the refrigerator and consume within 2 days for the best flavor.

Serving Size:

Makes approximately 8 servings (1 cup per serving)

Nutritional Information (per serving):

Calories: 0
Protein: 0g
Carbohydrates: 0g
Dietary Fiber: 0g
Sugars: 0g
Fat: 0g
Saturated Fat: 0g
Sodium: 0mg
Vitamin C: 4% DV (from lemon)
Calcium: 0% DV
Iron: 0% DV

17.5 Lavender Chamomile Tea

Ingredients:

- 1 tablespoon dried chamomile flowers
- 1 tablespoon dried lavender buds
- 4 cups water
- 1-2 teaspoons honey or maple syrup (optional, for sweetness)
- Lemon slices (optional, for garnish)

Directions:

1. Boil the Water: In a medium pot, bring 4 cups of water to a boil.

2. Add Chamomile and Lavender: Once the water is boiling, add the dried chamomile flowers and dried lavender buds. Reduce the heat and let it simmer for about 5-10 minutes.

3. Strain the Tea: After simmering, remove the pot from the heat. Strain the tea into a teapot or directly into cups to remove the chamomile flowers and lavender buds.

4. Add Sweetener (Optional): Stir in honey or maple syrup if desired.

5. Serve: Pour the tea into cups and enjoy it hot. Garnish with lemon slices if desired.

6. Store: Store any leftover tea in an airtight container in the refrigerator for up to 2 days. Reheat or serve chilled.

Serving Size:

Makes approximately 4 servings (1 cup per serving)
Nutritional Information (per serving, without optional ingredients):

Calories: 0
Protein: 0g
Carbohydrates: 0g
Dietary Fiber: 0g
Sugars: 0g
Fat: 0g
Saturated Fat: 0g
Sodium: 0mg
Vitamin C: 0% DV
Calcium: 0% DV
Iron: 0% DV

18. Smooth and Satisfying Drinks

18.1 Almond Milk Chai Latte

Ingredients:

- 2 cups unsweetened almond milk
- 2 black tea bags or 2 teaspoons loose black tea
- 1 cinnamon stick
- 4 whole cloves
- 4 whole cardamom pods, slightly crushed
- 1-inch piece of fresh ginger, sliced
- 1 teaspoon vanilla extract
- 1-2 tablespoons maple syrup or honey (optional, for sweetness)

Directions:

1. Heat the Milk: In a medium saucepan, heat the almond milk over medium heat until it starts to simmer. Do not let it boil.

2. Add Spices and Tea: Add the black tea bags (or loose tea), cinnamon stick, cloves, cardamom pods, and ginger slices to the simmering almond milk.

3. Simmer: Reduce the heat to low and let the mixture simmer for about 10 minutes, allowing the flavors to meld together.

4. Strain the Tea: After simmering, remove the saucepan from the heat. Strain the chai latte into a teapot or directly into cups to remove the tea bags and spices.

5. Add Vanilla and Sweetener (Optional): Stir in the vanilla extract and sweeten with maple syrup or honey if desired.

6. Serve: Pour the chai latte into mugs and enjoy it hot.

Serving Size:

Makes approximately 2 servings (1 cup per serving)
Nutritional Information (per serving, without optional ingredients):

Calories: 40
Protein: 1g
Carbohydrates: 2g
Dietary Fiber: 1g
Sugars: 0g
Fat: 3g
Saturated Fat: 0g
Sodium: 150mg
Calcium: 20% DV
Iron: 2% DV

18.2 Blueberry and Basil Smoothie

Ingredients:

- 1 cup fresh or frozen blueberries
- 1 banana
- 1 cup unsweetened almond milk (or any plant-based milk)
- 1/2 cup plain yogurt (dairy-free if needed)
- 1 tablespoon fresh basil leaves
- 1 tablespoon chia seeds
- 1 tablespoon honey or maple syrup (optional, for sweetness)
- 1/2 cup ice cubes (optional)

Directions:

1. Prepare Ingredients: If using fresh blueberries, wash them thoroughly. Peel the banana and gather all ingredients.

2. Blend: In a blender, combine the blueberries, banana, almond milk, yogurt, fresh basil leaves, chia seeds, and honey or maple syrup (if using).

3. Add Ice: If you prefer a colder, thicker smoothie, add the ice cubes to the blender.

4. Blend Until Smooth: Blend on high speed until the mixture is smooth and creamy.

5. Serve: Pour the smoothie into glasses and enjoy immediately.

Serving Size:

Makes approximately 2 servings (1 cup per serving)

Nutritional Information (per serving):

Calories: 150

Protein: 3g

Carbohydrates: 30g

Dietary Fiber: 6g

Sugars: 16g

Fat: 3g

Saturated Fat: 0g

Sodium: 85mg

Vitamin A: 2% DV

Vitamin C: 25% DV

Calcium: 15% DV

Iron: 6% DV

18.3 Golden Milk (Turmeric Latte)

Ingredients:

- 2 cups unsweetened almond milk (or any plant-based milk)
- 1 teaspoon ground turmeric
- 1/2 teaspoon ground cinnamon
- 1/4 teaspoon ground ginger (or 1/2 inch fresh ginger, grated)
- 1 tablespoon honey or maple syrup (optional, for sweetness)
- 1/2 teaspoon vanilla extract
- Pinch of black pepper
- Pinch of ground nutmeg (optional)
- Pinch of ground cardamom (optional)

Directions:

1. Heat the Milk: In a small saucepan, combine the almond milk, ground turmeric, ground cinnamon, ground ginger (or fresh ginger), and black pepper.

2. Simmer: Heat the mixture over medium heat, stirring frequently, until it begins to simmer. Do not let it boil.

3. Add Sweetener and Flavoring: Once the mixture is hot, remove it from the heat. Stir in the honey or maple syrup (if using) and vanilla extract. Add a pinch of ground nutmeg and cardamom if desired.

4. Strain (if using fresh ginger): If you used fresh ginger, strain the mixture through a fine mesh sieve into cups.

5. Serve: Pour the golden milk into mugs and enjoy it warm.

Serving Size:

Makes approximately 2 servings (1 cup per serving)

Nutritional Information (per serving, without optional ingredients):

Calories: 60

Protein: 1g

Carbohydrates: 9g

Dietary Fiber: 1g

Sugars: 6g

Fat: 2.5g

Saturated Fat: 0g

Sodium: 150mg

Vitamin A: 10% DV

Vitamin C: 0% DV

Calcium: 25% DV

Iron: 4% DV

18.4 Matcha Green Tea Smoothie

Ingredients:

- 1 teaspoon matcha green tea powder
- 1 cup unsweetened almond milk (or any plant-based milk)
- 1 frozen banana
- 1/2 cup spinach leaves
- 1/2 avocado
- 1 tablespoon chia seeds
- 1 tablespoon honey or maple syrup (optional, for sweetness)
- 1/2 cup ice cubes (optional)

Directions:

1. Prepare Ingredients: Gather all ingredients. Peel the banana and cut the avocado in half, removing the pit.

2. Blend: In a blender, combine the matcha green tea powder, almond milk, frozen banana, spinach leaves, avocado, chia seeds, and honey or maple syrup (if using).

3. Add Ice: If you prefer a colder, thicker smoothie, add the ice cubes to the blender.

4. Blend Until Smooth: Blend on high speed until the mixture is smooth and creamy.

5. Serve: Pour the smoothie into glasses and enjoy immediately.

Serving Size:

Makes approximately 2 servings (1 cup per serving)

Nutritional Information (per serving, without optional ingredients):

Calories: 170

Protein: 3g

Carbohydrates: 23g

Dietary Fiber: 7g

Sugars: 10g

Fat: 8g

Saturated Fat: 1g

Sodium: 80mg

Vitamin A: 20% DV

Vitamin C: 20% DV

Calcium: 20% DV

Iron: 8% DV

18.5 Spiced Apple Cider

Ingredients:

- 4 cups apple cider (preferably organic, no added sugars)
- 1 cinnamon stick
- 4 whole cloves
- 2 star anise pods
- 1/2 teaspoon ground nutmeg
- 1 orange, sliced
- 1 tablespoon maple syrup or honey (optional, for sweetness)

Directions:

1. Combine Ingredients: In a medium saucepan, combine the apple cider, cinnamon stick, cloves, star anise pods, ground nutmeg, and orange slices.

2. Heat the Cider: Place the saucepan over medium heat and bring the mixture to a simmer. Do not let it boil.

3. Simmer: Reduce the heat to low and let the cider simmer for about 20-30 minutes to allow the spices to infuse.

4. Strain the Cider: After simmering, remove the saucepan from the heat. Strain the cider through a fine mesh sieve into a teapot or directly into cups to remove the spices and orange slices.

5. Add Sweetener (Optional): Stir in the maple syrup or honey if desired.

6. Serve: Pour the spiced apple cider into mugs and enjoy it warm.

Serving Size:

Makes approximately 4 servings (1 cup per serving)
Nutritional Information (per serving, without optional ingredients):

Calories: 120
Protein: 0g
Carbohydrates: 30g
Dietary Fiber: 0g
Sugars: 24g
Fat: 0g
Saturated Fat: 0g
Sodium: 10mg
Vitamin A: 2% DV
Vitamin C: 6% DV
Calcium: 2% DV
Iron: 2% DV

Part IX: Special Diet Considerations

19. Gluten-Free and Low-Histamine

19.1 Buckwheat Pancakes

Ingredients:

- 1 cup buckwheat flour
- 1 tablespoon coconut sugar or honey (optional)
- 1 teaspoon baking powder
- 1/4 teaspoon baking soda
- 1/4 teaspoon salt
- 1 cup unsweetened almond milk (or any plant-based milk)
- 1 tablespoon apple cider vinegar
- 1 large egg (or flax egg for vegan option)
- 1 teaspoon vanilla extract
- 2 tablespoons coconut oil (melted) or olive oil
- Fresh berries and maple syrup for serving

Directions:

1. Prepare Wet Ingredients:

- In a small bowl, mix the almond milk and apple cider vinegar. Let it sit for 5 minutes to create a buttermilk substitute.
- In another bowl, whisk together the egg (or flax egg), vanilla extract, and melted coconut oil.

2. Combine Dry Ingredients:

- In a large mixing bowl, combine the buckwheat flour, coconut sugar (if using), baking powder, baking soda, and salt.

3. Mix Ingredients:

- Pour the wet ingredients into the dry ingredients. Mix until just combined. Do not overmix; the batter should be slightly lumpy.

4. Cook Pancakes:

- Heat a non-stick skillet or griddle over medium heat. Lightly grease with a little coconut oil or olive oil.
- Pour 1/4 cup of batter onto the skillet for each pancake. Cook until bubbles form on the surface and the edges look set, about 2-3 minutes.
- Flip the pancakes and cook for another 1-2 minutes, until golden brown.

5. Serve:

- Serve the pancakes warm with fresh berries and a drizzle of maple syrup.

Cooking Time:

Prep Time: 10 minutes
Cook Time: 15 minutes
Total Time: 25 minutes

Serving Size:

Makes approximately 8 pancakes

Nutritional Information (per pancake):

Calories: 80
Protein: 2g

Carbohydrates: 12g

Dietary Fiber: 2g

Sugars: 2g

Fat: 3g

Saturated Fat: 2g

Sodium: 150mg

Vitamin A: 0% DV

Vitamin C: 0% DV

Calcium: 4% DV

Iron: 4% DV

19.2 Gluten-Free Veggie Burgers

Ingredients:

- 1 cup cooked quinoa
- 1 can (15 oz) black beans, drained and rinsed
- 1/2 cup grated carrot
- 1/2 cup finely chopped bell pepper
- 1/4 cup finely chopped red onion
- 2 cloves garlic, minced
- 1/4 cup gluten-free oat flour (or ground oats)
- 1 tablespoon ground flaxseed
- 1 teaspoon cumin
- 1/2 teaspoon smoked paprika
- 1/2 teaspoon salt
- 1/4 teaspoon black pepper
- 2 tablespoons olive oil (for cooking)

Directions:

1. Prepare the Ingredients:

- Cook quinoa according to package instructions if not already done.
- Drain and rinse the black beans, then mash them in a large mixing bowl until mostly smooth with some chunks remaining.

2. Mix the Veggies and Spices:

- Add the grated carrot, chopped bell pepper, chopped red onion, minced garlic, oat flour, ground flaxseed, cumin, smoked paprika, salt, and black pepper to the mashed beans. Mix well.

3. Add Quinoa:

- Fold in the cooked quinoa until evenly distributed throughout the mixture.

4. Form Patties:

- Divide the mixture into 6 equal portions and shape each portion into a patty about 1/2 inch thick.

5. Preheat the Skillet:

- Heat 1 tablespoon of olive oil in a large non-stick skillet over medium heat.

6. Cook the Patties:

- Place the patties in the skillet and cook for 4-5 minutes on each side, or until they are golden brown and firm. You may need to cook them in batches, adding more oil as needed.

7. Serve:

- Serve the veggie burgers on gluten-free buns with your favorite toppings, such as lettuce, tomato, avocado, and a dollop of dairy-free sauce.

Cooking Time:

Prep Time: 15 minutes
Cook Time: 10 minutes per batch
Total Time: 25-35 minutes

Serving Size:

Makes approximately 6 veggie burgers

Nutritional Information (per burger, without bun and toppings):

Calories: 150

Protein: 5g

Carbohydrates: 20g

Dietary Fiber: 6g

Sugars: 2g

Fat: 6g

Saturated Fat: 1g

Sodium: 300mg

Vitamin A: 50% DV

Vitamin C: 30% DV

Calcium: 4% DV

Iron: 10% DV

19.3 Quinoa and Spinach Stuffed Mushrooms

Ingredients:

- 12 large portobello or cremini mushrooms, stems removed and cleaned
- 1 cup cooked quinoa
- 1 tablespoon olive oil
- 1 small onion, finely chopped
- 2 cloves garlic, minced
- 3 cups fresh spinach, chopped
- 1/4 cup nutritional yeast (for a cheesy flavor, optional)
- 1/4 cup finely chopped fresh parsley
- 1 teaspoon dried oregano
- 1/2 teaspoon salt
- 1/4 teaspoon black pepper
- 1/4 cup gluten-free breadcrumbs (optional)
- 2 tablespoons olive oil (for drizzling)

Directions:

1. Preheat Oven:

- Preheat your oven to 375°F (190°C).

2. Prepare the Mushroom Caps:

- Clean the mushroom caps with a damp cloth. Remove and finely chop the stems, setting them aside for the stuffing.

3. Cook the Aromatics:

- In a large skillet, heat 1 tablespoon of olive oil over medium heat. Add the chopped onion and cook for 3-4 minutes until it becomes translucent.

- Add the minced garlic and cook for another minute until fragrant.

4. Add Spinach and Mushroom Stems:

- Add the chopped mushroom stems and cook for 2-3 minutes until softened.
- Add the chopped spinach and cook until wilted, about 2-3 minutes.

5. Combine with Quinoa:

- Transfer the cooked vegetables to a large bowl. Add the cooked quinoa, nutritional yeast (if using), chopped parsley, dried oregano, salt, and black pepper. Mix well to combine.

6. Stuff the Mushrooms:

- Spoon the quinoa and spinach mixture into each mushroom cap, packing it in firmly.
- If using, sprinkle the gluten-free breadcrumbs on top of the stuffed mushrooms.

7. Bake:

- Place the stuffed mushrooms on a baking sheet. Drizzle with 2 tablespoons of olive oil.
- Bake in the preheated oven for 20-25 minutes, or until the mushrooms are tender and the tops are golden brown.

8. Serve:

- Serve the stuffed mushrooms warm, garnished with additional fresh parsley if desired.

Serving Size:

Makes approximately 4 servings (3 stuffed mushrooms per serving)

Nutritional Information (per serving, without optional ingredients):

Calories: 180

Protein: 6g

Carbohydrates: 20g

Dietary Fiber: 4g

Sugars: 3g

Fat: 8g

Saturated Fat: 1g

Sodium: 400mg

Vitamin A: 50% DV

Vitamin C: 25% DV

Calcium: 6% DV

Iron: 15% DV

19.4 Gluten-Free Lentil Loaf

Ingredients:

- 1 cup green or brown lentils, rinsed
- 2 1/2 cups water
- 1 tablespoon olive oil
- 1 small onion, finely chopped
- 2 cloves garlic, minced
- 1 cup grated carrot
- 1 cup finely chopped celery
- 1/2 cup rolled oats (gluten-free)
- 1/2 cup gluten-free breadcrumbs
- 2 tablespoons ground flaxseed mixed with 6 tablespoons water (flax egg)
- 2 tablespoons tomato paste
- 1 tablespoon soy sauce (gluten-free)
- 1 teaspoon dried thyme
- 1 teaspoon dried oregano
- 1/2 teaspoon smoked paprika
- 1/2 teaspoon salt
- 1/4 teaspoon black pepper
- 1/4 cup ketchup (for topping, optional)

Directions:

1. Preheat your oven to 350°F (175°C).

2. In a medium pot, bring the lentils and water to a boil. Reduce the heat and simmer for about 25 minutes, or until the lentils are tender and the water is absorbed. Drain any excess water if necessary.

3. In a large skillet, heat the olive oil over medium heat. Add the chopped onion and cook for 3-4 minutes until translucent. Add the minced garlic and cook for another minute.

4. Stir in the grated carrot and chopped celery. Cook for an additional 5 minutes until the vegetables are tender.

5. In a large bowl, combine the cooked lentils, sautéed vegetables, rolled oats, gluten-free breadcrumbs, flax egg, tomato paste, soy sauce, dried thyme, dried oregano, smoked paprika, salt, and black pepper. Mix well until all ingredients are thoroughly combined.

6. Transfer the mixture into a parchment-lined loaf pan, pressing it down firmly to pack it tightly. If desired, spread the ketchup on top for a glaze.

7. Bake in the preheated oven for 45-50 minutes, or until the loaf is firm and golden brown on top.

8. Allow the loaf to cool in the pan for 10-15 minutes before slicing and serving.

Cooking Time:

Prep Time: 20 minutes
Cook Time: 45-50 minutes
Total Time: 1 hour 10 minutes
Serving Size: Makes approximately 8 servings

Nutritional Information (per serving):

Calories: 200

Protein: 8g

Carbohydrates: 30g

Dietary Fiber: 8g

Sugars: 4g

Fat: 5g

Saturated Fat: 1g

Sodium: 400mg

Vitamin A: 50% DV

Vitamin C: 10% DV

Calcium: 6% DV

Iron: 15% DV

19.5 Rice and Veggie Stuffed Cabbage Rolls

Ingredients:

- 1 large head of cabbage
- 1 cup cooked rice (white or brown)
- 1 tablespoon olive oil
- 1 small onion, finely chopped
- 2 cloves garlic, minced
- 1 carrot, grated
- 1 zucchini, grated
- 1 cup mushrooms, finely chopped
- 1/2 cup cooked lentils (optional for extra protein)
- 1 teaspoon dried thyme
- 1 teaspoon dried oregano
- 1/2 teaspoon smoked paprika
- 1/2 teaspoon salt
- 1/4 teaspoon black pepper
- 1 can (15 ounces) diced tomatoes, no added salt
- 1 cup tomato sauce (low-histamine if available)
- Fresh parsley for garnish

Directions:

1. Preheat your oven to 350°F (175°C).

2. In a large pot, bring water to a boil. Carefully remove the core from the cabbage and place the whole head into the boiling water. Cook for 2-3 minutes, or until the outer leaves begin to soften and peel away easily. Remove the leaves and repeat until you have 12 large leaves. Set aside to cool.

3. In a large skillet, heat the olive oil over medium heat. Add the chopped onion and cook for 3-4 minutes until translucent. Add the minced garlic and cook for another minute.

4. Stir in the grated carrot, grated zucchini, and chopped mushrooms. Cook for an additional 5 minutes until the vegetables are tender and any excess moisture has evaporated.

5. In a large bowl, combine the cooked rice, cooked lentils (if using), sautéed vegetables, dried thyme, dried oregano, smoked paprika, salt, and black pepper. Mix well to combine.

6. Lay each cabbage leaf flat and place a few spoonfuls of the rice and veggie mixture in the center. Fold the sides over the filling and roll up tightly.

7. In a large baking dish, spread half of the diced tomatoes and half of the tomato sauce on the bottom.

8. Arrange the cabbage rolls seam side down in the baking dish. Pour the remaining diced tomatoes and tomato sauce over the top.

9. Cover the dish with aluminum foil and bake in the preheated oven for 45-50 minutes, or until the cabbage is tender and the filling is heated through.

10. Remove from the oven and let cool for a few minutes before serving. Garnish with fresh parsley.

Serving Size: Makes approximately 4 servings (3 cabbage rolls per serving)

Nutritional Information (per serving):

Calories: 220

Protein: 7g

Carbohydrates: 36g

Dietary Fiber: 8g

Sugars: 8g

Fat: 6g

Saturated Fat: 1g

Sodium: 400mg

Vitamin A: 60% DV

Vitamin C: 70% DV

Calcium: 10% DV

Iron: 15% DV

20. Low-Carb and Low-Histamine

20.1 Cauliflower Rice Stir-Fry

Ingredients:

- 1 head of cauliflower, grated into rice-like texture
- 1 tablespoon sesame oil
- 1 small onion, thinly sliced
- 2 cloves garlic, minced
- 1 bell pepper, thinly sliced
- 1 carrot, thinly sliced or grated
- 1 cup broccoli florets
- 1 cup snap peas, trimmed
- 1/2 cup frozen edamame, thawed
- 2 tablespoons low-sodium soy sauce (gluten-free if needed)
- 1 tablespoon rice vinegar
- 1 teaspoon fresh ginger, grated
- 1/2 teaspoon sriracha or chili paste (optional)
- Salt and pepper to taste
- Fresh cilantro or green onions for garnish

Directions:

1. Prepare the Cauliflower Rice:

- Remove the core from the cauliflower and grate it using a box grater or pulse it in a food processor until it resembles rice grains. Set aside.

2. Stir-Fry:

- Heat sesame oil in a large skillet or wok over medium-high heat.

- Add the sliced onion and minced garlic, stirring constantly for 1-2 minutes until fragrant.

3. Add Vegetables:

- Add the bell pepper, carrot, broccoli florets, snap peas, and thawed edamame to the skillet. Stir-fry for 5-6 minutes until the vegetables are tender-crisp.

4. Incorporate Cauliflower Rice:

- Push the vegetables to one side of the skillet and add the grated cauliflower rice to the empty space.
- Stir-fry the cauliflower rice for 3-4 minutes until it starts to soften and becomes tender.

5. Seasoning:

- In a small bowl, mix together soy sauce, rice vinegar, grated ginger, and sriracha or chili paste (if using).
- Pour the sauce over the stir-fry and toss everything together until well combined. Cook for another 1-2 minutes to heat through.

6. Serve:

- Remove from heat and season with salt and pepper to taste.
- Garnish with fresh cilantro or green onions before serving.

Cooking Time:

Prep Time: 15 minutes

Cook Time: 10 minutes

Total Time: 25 minutes

Serving Size: Makes approximately 4 servings

Nutritional Information (per serving):

Calories: 150

Protein: 8g

Carbohydrates: 20g

Dietary Fiber: 8g

Sugars: 8g

Fat: 6g

Saturated Fat: 1g

Sodium: 400mg

Vitamin A: 120% DV

Vitamin C: 160% DV

Calcium: 8% DV

Iron: 15% DV

20.2 Zucchini Lasagna

Ingredients:

- 4 medium zucchinis, thinly sliced lengthwise
- 2 cups marinara sauce (store-bought or homemade)
- 1 cup ricotta cheese (or dairy-free alternative)
- 1 cup spinach, chopped
- 1 cup mushrooms, sliced
- 1 bell pepper, diced
- 1 small onion, diced
- 2 cloves garlic, minced
- 1 tablespoon olive oil
- 1 teaspoon dried oregano
- 1 teaspoon dried basil
- Salt and pepper to taste
- 1/2 cup shredded mozzarella cheese (or dairy-free alternative)
- Fresh basil leaves for garnish

Directions:

1. Prepare the Zucchini:

- Preheat oven to 375°F (190°C).
- Slice the zucchinis lengthwise into thin strips using a mandoline slicer or a sharp knife. Lay them out on paper towels and sprinkle with salt. Let them sit for 10 minutes to release excess moisture, then pat dry with paper towels.

2. Prepare the Filling:

- Heat olive oil in a large skillet over medium heat. Add onion and garlic, sauté until fragrant, about 2 minutes.

- Add mushrooms, bell pepper, dried oregano, dried basil, salt, and pepper. Cook until vegetables are tender, about 5-7 minutes.
- Stir in spinach and cook until wilted, about 2 minutes. Remove from heat and set aside.

3. Assemble the Lasagna:

- Spread a thin layer of marinara sauce on the bottom of a 9x13-inch baking dish.
- Arrange a layer of zucchini slices over the sauce.
- Spread half of the ricotta cheese evenly over the zucchini slices.
- Spoon half of the vegetable mixture over the ricotta cheese.
- Repeat with another layer of marinara sauce, zucchini slices, ricotta cheese, and vegetables.

4. Bake:

- Top with shredded mozzarella cheese.
- Cover the baking dish with foil and bake in the preheated oven for 30 minutes.
- Remove the foil and bake uncovered for an additional 10 minutes or until the cheese is bubbly and golden.

5. Serve:

- Remove from the oven and let it cool for 10 minutes before slicing.
- Garnish with fresh basil leaves before serving.

Cooking Time:

Prep Time: 20 minutes

Cook Time: 40 minutes

Total Time: 1 hour

Serving Size: Makes approximately 6 servings

Nutritional Information (per serving):

Calories: 220
Protein: 12g
Carbohydrates: 18g
Dietary Fiber: 4g
Sugars: 8g
Fat: 12g
Saturated Fat: 4g
Cholesterol: 20mg
Sodium: 480mg
Vitamin A: 40% DV
Vitamin C: 60% DV
Calcium: 25% DV
Iron: 10% DV

20.3 Spaghetti Squash with Pesto

Ingredients:

- 1 medium spaghetti squash
- 2 cups fresh basil leaves
- 1/2 cup grated Parmesan cheese (or nutritional yeast for vegan option)
- 1/3 cup pine nuts, toasted
- 2 cloves garlic, minced
- 1/2 cup extra-virgin olive oil
- Salt and pepper to taste
- Cherry tomatoes, halved, for garnish (optional)

Directions:

1. Prepare the Spaghetti Squash:

- Preheat oven to 400°F (200°C).
- Cut the spaghetti squash in half lengthwise and scoop out the seeds with a spoon.
- Drizzle the cut sides with olive oil and sprinkle with salt and pepper.
- Place squash halves cut side down on a baking sheet lined with parchment paper. Roast for 35-45 minutes, or until tender and easily pierced with a fork.
- Let the squash cool slightly, then use a fork to scrape the flesh into strands. Place the strands in a large bowl.

2. Prepare the Pesto:

- In a food processor, combine basil leaves, Parmesan cheese (or nutritional yeast), pine nuts, and minced garlic.
- Pulse until coarsely chopped.
- With the food processor running, slowly add the olive oil in a steady stream until the pesto is smooth and well combined.

- Season with salt and pepper to taste.

3. Combine and Serve:

- Add the prepared pesto to the bowl of spaghetti squash strands.
- Toss gently until the squash is evenly coated with pesto.
- Divide the spaghetti squash into serving bowls.
- Garnish with cherry tomatoes, if desired.

Cooking Time:

Prep Time: 15 minutes

Cook Time: 40 minutes

Total Time: 55 minutes

Serving Size: Makes approximately 4 servings

Nutritional Information (per serving):

Calories: 350

Protein: 7g

Carbohydrates: 18g

Dietary Fiber: 4g

Sugars: 6g

Fat: 30g

Saturated Fat: 5g

Cholesterol: 5mg

Sodium: 250mg

Vitamin A: 40% DV

Vitamin C: 20% DV

Calcium: 20% DV

Iron: 15% DV

20.4 Eggplant Rollatini

Ingredients:

- 2 medium eggplants, sliced lengthwise into 1/4-inch thick slices
- 2 cups ricotta cheese (or dairy-free alternative)
- 1 cup grated Parmesan cheese (or nutritional yeast for vegan option), divided
- 1 cup shredded mozzarella cheese (or dairy-free alternative), divided
- 2 cups marinara sauce (store-bought or homemade)
- 2 cloves garlic, minced
- 1 tablespoon olive oil
- 1 teaspoon dried oregano
- 1 teaspoon dried basil
- Salt and pepper to taste
- Fresh basil leaves for garnish

Directions:

1. Prepare the Eggplant:

- Preheat oven to 400°F (200°C).
- Place eggplant slices on a baking sheet lined with parchment paper.
- Drizzle olive oil over the eggplant slices and season with salt and pepper.
- Roast in the preheated oven for 15-20 minutes, flipping halfway through, until tender and lightly browned. Remove from oven and let cool.

2. Prepare the Filling:

- In a medium bowl, combine ricotta cheese, half of the grated Parmesan cheese, half of the shredded mozzarella cheese, minced garlic, dried oregano, dried basil, salt, and pepper. Mix well.

3. Assemble the Rollatini:

- Spread a thin layer of marinara sauce on the bottom of a 9x13-inch baking dish.
- Place a spoonful of the ricotta mixture onto each eggplant slice and roll it up. Place each rollatini seam-side down in the baking dish.

4. Bake:

- Pour the remaining marinara sauce over the eggplant rollatini.
- Sprinkle the remaining grated Parmesan cheese and shredded mozzarella cheese over the top.
- Cover the baking dish with foil and bake in the preheated oven for 25 minutes.
- Remove the foil and bake uncovered for an additional 10 minutes or until the cheese is melted and bubbly.

5. Serve:

- Remove from the oven and let it cool for 5-10 minutes before serving.
- Garnish with fresh basil leaves before serving.

Cooking Time:

Prep Time: 20 minutes

Cook Time: 35 minutes

Total Time: 55 minutes

Serving Size: Makes approximately 6 servings

Nutritional Information (per serving):

Calories: 350

Protein: 20g

Carbohydrates: 20g

Dietary Fiber: 6g

Sugars: 10g

Fat: 22g

Saturated Fat: 10g

Cholesterol: 50mg

Sodium: 900mg

Vitamin A: 25% DV

Vitamin C: 15% DV

Calcium: 40% DV

Iron: 10% DV

20.5 Cauliflower Pizza Crust with Veggie Toppings

Ingredients:

- 1 medium head cauliflower, grated (about 4 cups)
- 1/2 cup shredded mozzarella cheese (or dairy-free alternative)
- 1/4 cup grated Parmesan cheese (or nutritional yeast for vegan option)
- 1 teaspoon dried oregano
- 1/2 teaspoon garlic powder
- 1/4 teaspoon salt
- 1/4 teaspoon black pepper
- 1 egg (or flaxseed meal for vegan option)
- 1/2 cup marinara sauce (store-bought or homemade)
- 1 cup assorted veggies (such as bell peppers, mushrooms, spinach, and cherry tomatoes), chopped
- 1/2 cup shredded mozzarella cheese (or dairy-free alternative), for topping
- Fresh basil leaves for garnish

Directions:

1. Prepare the Cauliflower Crust:

- Preheat oven to 425°F (220°C). Line a baking sheet with parchment paper.
- Grate the cauliflower using a box grater or food processor until you have about 4 cups of cauliflower crumbles.
- Place the grated cauliflower in a microwave-safe bowl and microwave on high for 5-6 minutes, until soft. Let it cool for a few minutes.
- Transfer the cauliflower to a clean kitchen towel or cheesecloth. Squeeze out as much liquid as possible.

- In a mixing bowl, combine the drained cauliflower, shredded mozzarella cheese, grated Parmesan cheese, dried oregano, garlic powder, salt, pepper, and egg (or flaxseed meal). Mix well.

2. Form the Crust:

- Transfer the cauliflower mixture to the prepared baking sheet. Using your hands, flatten and shape the mixture into a thin, round crust about 1/4-inch thick.

3. Bake the Crust:

- Bake in the preheated oven for 15-20 minutes, or until the crust is golden and firm to the touch.

4. Prepare the Pizza:

- Spread marinara sauce evenly over the baked cauliflower crust.
- Top with chopped assorted veggies and shredded mozzarella cheese (or dairy-free alternative).

5. Bake Again:

- Return the pizza to the oven and bake for an additional 10-15 minutes, or until the cheese is melted and bubbly.

6. Serve:

- Remove from the oven and let it cool for a few minutes before slicing.
- Garnish with fresh basil leaves before serving.

Cooking Time:

Prep Time: 20 minutes

Cook Time: 35 minutes

Total Time: 55 minutes

Serving Size: Makes 1 large pizza (about 8 slices)

Nutritional Information (per slice):

Calories: 120
Protein: 8g
Carbohydrates: 10g
Dietary Fiber: 3g
Sugars: 4g
Fat: 6g
Saturated Fat: 3g
Cholesterol: 30mg
Sodium: 320mg
Vitamin A: 15% DV
Vitamin C: 45% DV
Calcium: 20% DV
Iron: 5% DV

Conclusion

21. Living Well with Histamine Intolerance

21.1 Tips for Dining Out

Dining out with histamine intolerance can be challenging, but with careful planning and communication, you can still enjoy meals at restaurants. Here are some practical tips to help you navigate dining out while managing histamine intolerance:

1. Research Restaurants in Advance:

- Look for restaurants that offer fresh, made-to-order dishes rather than pre-prepared foods.
- Check online menus to see if they offer low-histamine options or customizable dishes.
- Read reviews and look for feedback from other diners with dietary restrictions.

2. Communicate Clearly with Staff:

- Call the restaurant ahead of time to inform them of your histamine intolerance and ask if they can accommodate your needs.
- Speak directly to the chef or manager if possible, as they will have the most control over ingredients and preparation methods.
- Clearly explain your dietary restrictions to the server when you arrive.

3. Ask About Ingredients and Preparation Methods:

- Inquire about the ingredients used in dishes, especially sauces, marinades, and dressings, which may contain high-histamine items.

- Ask how dishes are prepared, focusing on freshness and avoidance of aged, fermented, or preserved ingredients.
- Request that your meal be cooked without high-histamine spices like soy sauce, vinegar, or fish sauce.

4. Opt for Simple, Fresh Dishes:

- Choose dishes that are likely to be made with fresh, whole ingredients such as salads, steamed vegetables, and grilled proteins.
- Avoid dishes with aged cheeses, cured meats, or fermented foods.
- Select plain options for sides, like rice or potatoes, which are less likely to contain hidden histamines.

5. Customizing Your Order:

- Don't hesitate to ask for modifications to your meal to avoid high-histamine ingredients.
- Request dressings and sauces on the side so you can control the amount you consume or avoid them altogether.
- Ask for freshly cooked proteins, specifying that they be prepared without marinades or seasoning mixes that could contain histamines.

6. Carry a List of Safe Foods and Ingredients:

- Keep a list of low-histamine foods and ingredients with you to help guide your choices.
- Use the list to quickly check menu items and ensure they align with your dietary needs.

7. Be Prepared with Snacks:

- Bring your own low-histamine snacks in case the restaurant cannot fully accommodate your needs.

- Having a safe snack on hand can help you avoid hunger and frustration if suitable options are limited.

8. Choose Restaurants with Flexibility:

- Favor establishments that are known for accommodating dietary restrictions and have a reputation for good customer service.
- Ethnic cuisines that rely on fresh ingredients, like Japanese (sushi without soy sauce) or Mediterranean, can often be more accommodating to low-histamine diets.

9. Trust Your Instincts:

- If a restaurant seems unable or unwilling to accommodate your dietary needs, it's okay to leave and find a more suitable option.
- Your health and well-being are the top priority, so don't feel obligated to stay in an environment that feels risky.

By following these tips, you can enjoy dining out while managing histamine intolerance. With preparation and clear communication, you can minimize the risk of histamine reactions and still have a pleasant dining experience.

21.2 Maintaining Balance and Wellness

1. Prioritize Whole Foods:

- Focus on a diet rich in fresh, whole foods like fruits, vegetables, whole grains, nuts, and seeds. These foods are less likely to contain hidden histamines and provide essential nutrients for overall health.
- Avoid processed foods, which often contain additives, preservatives, and hidden ingredients that can trigger histamine release.

2. Stay Hydrated:

- Drink plenty of water throughout the day to help your body manage histamine levels and maintain overall health.
- Herbal teas and infused waters are excellent choices, but be mindful of any potential histamine triggers.

3. Manage Stress:

- Chronic stress can exacerbate histamine intolerance. Incorporate stress-reducing practices into your daily routine, such as yoga, meditation, deep breathing exercises, or spending time in nature.
- Regular physical activity, like walking or gentle exercise, can also help manage stress levels.

4. Get Adequate Sleep:

- Aim for 7-9 hours of quality sleep per night to support overall health and help your body manage histamine levels.
- Establish a consistent sleep schedule and create a relaxing bedtime routine to improve sleep quality.

5. Exercise Regularly:

- Engage in regular physical activity to support overall health and wellness. Exercise can help regulate histamine levels and improve your immune system.
- Choose activities that you enjoy, such as walking, swimming, cycling, or yoga, and aim for at least 150 minutes of moderate-intensity exercise per week.

6. Support Gut Health:

- A healthy gut microbiome is crucial for managing histamine intolerance. Include probiotic-rich foods like low-histamine fermented foods, or consider a probiotic supplement, to support gut health.
- Avoid high-histamine fermented foods like sauerkraut, kimchi, and certain yogurts.

7. Monitor Your Symptoms:

- Keep a detailed food diary to track your symptoms and identify any patterns or triggers. Note the foods you eat, the time of consumption, and any symptoms you experience.
- Use this information to make informed decisions about your diet and lifestyle.

8. Supplement Wisely:

- Some supplements can help manage histamine levels and support overall health. Vitamin C, quercetin, and bromelain are known for their antihistamine properties.
- Always consult with a healthcare provider before starting any new supplements to ensure they are safe and appropriate for you.

9. Connect with a Healthcare Professional:

- Work with a healthcare professional, such as a nutritionist or dietitian, who specializes in histamine intolerance. They can help you develop a personalized plan to manage your condition.
- Regular check-ups and open communication with your healthcare provider can ensure you are on the right track and making necessary adjustments.

10. Cultivate a Positive Mindset:

- Managing histamine intolerance can be challenging, but maintaining a positive outlook can significantly impact your overall well-being.
- Surround yourself with supportive friends and family, and engage in activities that bring you joy and fulfillment.

Maintaining balance and wellness while managing histamine intolerance requires a holistic approach. By prioritizing whole foods, staying hydrated, managing stress, getting adequate sleep, exercising regularly, supporting gut health, monitoring symptoms, supplementing wisely, connecting with healthcare professionals, and cultivating a positive mindset, you can effectively manage your condition and improve your overall quality of life.

www.ingramcontent.com/pod-product-compliance
Lightning Source LLC
Chambersburg PA
CBHW081209260726
48653CB00010BA/3576